Challenging Cases in Geriatric Medicine

Geriatric medicine is challenging. People present with multiple problems at the same time, and case studies provide a good way to discuss this complexity. This book describes 30 cases of older people with frailty presenting to acute medical services. They cover a wide range of common presentations and management issues and explore the interplay of acute illness, multi-morbidity, and physical and cognitive impairments. The book focuses on medicine optimisation, shared decision-making, and advance care planning using key test results and imaging studies. Management options are discussed where disease-specific guidelines may not provide the solution when treating older adults.

Key Features:

- Provides real-world complex examples with consequent nuanced decision-making.
- Uses case studies to address interactions of acute illnesses, polypharmacy, and physical and cognitive impairments for clinicians and trainees in geriatric and general internal medicine and general practitioners.
- Discusses patient-centred management—balance of risks and benefits of different options, including shared decision-making and advance care planning.

Challenging Cases in Geriatric Medicine

Henry J Woodford and Francis J A Collin

CRC Press

Taylor & Francis Group

Boca Raton London New York

CRC Press is an imprint of the
Taylor & Francis Group, an **informa** business

Designed cover image: Shutterstock image id: 2212617371

First edition published 2026
by CRC Press
2385 NW Executive Center Drive, Suite 320, Boca Raton FL 33431

and by CRC Press
4 Park Square, Milton Park, Abingdon, Oxon, OX14 4RN

CRC Press is an imprint of Taylor & Francis Group, LLC

ISBN: 978-1-032-94847-8 (hbk)
ISBN: 978-1-032-94846-1 (pbk)
ISBN: 978-1-003-58200-7 (ebk)

DOI: 10.1201/9781003582007

Typeset in Minion
by Apex CoVantage, LLC

*With enormous thanks for the love and support
from our wives and children*

Ellie, Matilda, and Evie; Louise, Albert, and Ursula

Contents

Foreword

Doctors who choose to train in geriatric medicine are not afraid of complexity; it's often the challenge of solving a difficult puzzle that first attracts them to the specialty. Geriatricians—and the nurses and therapists with whom we work—know that algorithmic medicine doesn't work for older people, whose diagnoses may be legion and in whom successful management demands more than following a simple pathway. But it is difficult!

This tremendous book contains the stories of 30 patients. Each case is recognisable. There are familiar presentations: non-specific symptoms, anxious or absent families, beloved cats. Short vignettes paint vivid and engaging pictures. The authors offer sound advice on comprehensive assessment, tips for communication, and validated tools to help quantify issues with cognition or frailty. They accompany the reader through a maze of investigations and polypharmacy, highlighting interventions that add value and explaining why some tests or treatments are better discarded. At every turn, there is respect for the person at the centre of the story, and the authors' light touch guides the reader to an understanding of what matters most for each of their complex patients.

With wise and practical pointers, each chapter addresses the whole 'biopsychosocial' entity. If you're an established practitioner of the art of geriatric medicine, you will find both the known and the new in these pages. If you're setting out on your career, this book is an essential companion.

Lucy Pollock

Preface

This is a book of case scenarios of older people with frailty and multi-morbidity who have developed additional health problems. Their care is complex, and this book explores the key issues and resulting clinical decisions. The people described in this book are not real, but aspects of each are based on people we have met in hospitals and out-patient clinics, and so, hopefully, the characters will sound familiar to those who work with older people in healthcare settings. The use of cases enables discussion of multi-morbidity management in a way that standard textbooks do not. This is our rationale for creating this book. We have tried to put cases that discuss the foundations of geriatric medicine towards the start—i.e. comprehensive geriatric assessment, cognitive impairment, falls, mental capacity, advance care planning, and polypharmacy. Later chapters build on these foundations and introduce new clinical dilemmas.

This isn't a book about rare diseases or unusual presentations, quite the opposite. Common conditions are described presenting in common ways, i.e. older people with multi-morbidity, polypharmacy, and frailty who come into hospitals every day of the week. We have tried to select cases that help cover a broad range of common problems. Part of what makes geriatric medicine both challenging and rewarding is the complex blend of issues, which requires a person-centred approach involving a whole multidisciplinary team. We hope that this will shine out from our text.

Older people with frailty often present with multiple problems at once, including medication adverse effects, and in the context of functional impairment and limited life expectancy. These people are often excluded from clinical trials to test the efficacy, and safety, of medications. We don't have all the answers. This evidence-free zone is navigated with shared decision-making and by individualising care—what matters to you? Guideline-based prescribing is impersonal and unlikely to meet their needs, which is an example of modern medicine hitting the target but missing the point. We will suggest how medications can be optimised to achieve an individual's goals, sometimes through deprescribing. We will also explore advance care planning and end-of-life care. Our work is situated within the National Health Service in the UK and is determined by our local legal and ethical frameworks, which may differ in other locations.

We thank the remarkable patients that we have had the privilege to meet over the years for all that they have taught us and hope that we can be instrumental in providing the high-quality care that they deserve.

About the Authors

Dr Henry J Woodford was born in York and trained in medicine at King's College London. He is currently employed as a consultant geriatrician at Northumbria Healthcare in the northeast of England. He has a particular interest in medicine optimisation for older people and is the current chair of the relevant British Geriatrics Society special interest group. His publications include the textbooks *Essential Geriatrics* and coauthoring *Geriatric Medicine: 300 Specialty Certificate Exam Questions*. Outside of work, he tries to keep fit through circuit training, running, and indoor bouldering.

Dr Francis J A Collin was born in Nottingham and trained in medicine at the University of Bristol. He works as a consultant geriatrician at Northumbria Healthcare and has a particular interest in liaison working having worked as an orthogeriatrician and set up surgical geriatrics and community-based intermediate care services. Outside of work, he is a husband and father to two wonderful children and still plays Ultimate Frisbee internationally, having represented Great Britain.

Abbreviations

AAA	Abdominal aortic aneurysm	**HFrEF**	Heart failure with reduced ejection fraction
ACEi	ACE inhibitor		
ACS	Acute coronary syndrome	**ICD**	Implanted cardiac defibrillator
ADR	Adverse drug reaction		
AF	Atrial fibrillation	**ICH**	Intracranial haemorrhage
ARNI	Angiotensin receptor blocker and neprilysin inhibitor	**JVP**	Jugular venous pressure
		LABA	Long-acting beta 2 agonist
ARR	Absolute risk reduction	**LAMA**	Long-acting muscarinic antagonist
BB	Beta blocker		
bd	Twice daily	**LTOT**	Long-term oxygen therapy
BNP	B-type natriuretic peptide	**MCV**	Mean corpuscular volume
BP	Blood pressure	**MDI**	Multi-dose inhaler
BPH	Benign prostatic hyperplasia	**MR**	Modified release
bpm	Beats per minute	**MRA**	Mineralocorticoid receptor antagonist
BPSD	Behavioural and psychological symptoms of dementia		
		MRI	Magnetic resonance imaging
CAA	Cerebral amyloid angiopathy	**MSA**	Multiple system atrophy
CFS	Clinical Frailty Scale	**n**	At night
CGA	Comprehensive geriatric assessment	**NG**	Nasogastric
		NICE	National Institute for Health and Care Excellence
CLTI	Critical limb-threatening ischaemia		
		NNT	Number need to treat
COPD	Chronic obstructive pulmonary disease	**NSAID**	Non-steroidal anti-inflammatory drug
CPPD	Calcium pyrophosphate deposition disease	**NSTEMI**	Non-ST elevation myocardial infarct
CRP	C-reactive protein	**OA**	Osteoarthritis
CT	Computerised tomography	**od**	Once daily
D2A	Discharge to assess	**OH**	Orthostatic hypotension
DEXA	Dual-energy X-ray absorptiometry	**OSA**	Obstructive sleep apnoea
		PD	Parkinson's disease
DLB	Dementia with Lewy bodies	pO_2	Partial pressure of oxygen
DOAC	Direct oral anticoagulant	**PSP**	Progressive supranuclear palsy
DPI	Dry powder inhaler	**qds**	Four times daily
ECG	Electrocardiogram	**RA**	Rheumatoid arthritis
EF	Ejection fraction	**RRR**	Relative risk reduction
GI	Gastrointestinal	**SDH**	Subdural haematoma
HFmrEF	Heart failure with mildly reduced ejection fraction	**SGLT2i**	Sodium-glucose co-transporter 2 inhibitor
HFpEF	Heart failure with preserved ejection fraction	**SIADH**	Syndrome of inappropriate antidiuretic hormone secretion

SLT	Speech and language therapy	**T2DM**	Type 2 diabetes
SPECT	Single-photon emission computed tomography	**tds**	Three times daily
		TIA	Transient ischaemic attack
SSRI	Selective serotonin reuptake inhibitor	**TSH**	Thyroid-stimulating hormone
		UTI	Urinary tract infection
STEMI	ST-elevation myocardial infarct	**WCC**	White blood cell count

Case 1

Clive

Clive is an 89-year-old retired decorator, who is seen in the emergency department. He had a fall around midnight in his bathroom at home while on the way to the toilet to pass urine. He thinks the fall was due to a simple trip and doesn't report any warning symptoms or loss of consciousness. He has not fallen over before. He was incontinent of urine while stuck on the floor. After a while, he was able to crawl to the telephone and called for help. He has some soreness in his left shoulder and buttock since the fall. He usually gets up twice during the night to pass urine. He has some mild chronic back pain. He was feeling reasonably well prior to the fall and has not noticed any other new symptoms.

Past Medical History

Hypertension
Osteoarthritis
Type 2 diabetes
Mild cognitive impairment

Social History

Clive lives alone, since his wife died, in a three-bedroom house. He is usually independent except for some help from his son to do his grocery shopping. He uses a stick to walk outdoors but tends to furniture walk indoors. There is a single banister rail on his staircase. He doesn't smoke or drink any alcohol.

Medication

Clopidogrel 75 mg od Metformin 500 mg bd Simvastatin 40 mg n	Gliclazide 40 mg bd Ramipril 5 mg od

Examination

Clive smells of urine. Heart sounds are normal. His chest is clear. There is no peripheral oedema. His abdomen is soft, suprapubic tenderness is noted, and bowel sounds are present. There are superficial grazes on both of his knees. His arms and legs move okay without any pain.

DOI: 10.1201/9781003582007-1

Blood pressure 134/68 mmHg, pulse 73 beats per minute, temperature 36.2°C, oxygen saturation 95% on air, glucose 6.3 mmol/L

Investigations

Biochemistry	Value	Reference range	Haematology	Value	Reference range
Sodium	141	133–146 mmol/L	Haemoglobin	134	130–180 g/L
Potassium	4.2	3.5–5.3 mmol/L	MCV	86	82–100 fL
Urea	6.7	2.5–7.8 mmol/L	White cell count	7.6	4–11 10⁹/L
Creatinine	71	64–104 umol/L	Platelets	233	140–400 10⁹/L
C-reactive protein	9	< 5 mg/L			

Hb_{A1C} 43 mmol/mol when last tested six weeks ago
ECG—79 bpm sinus rhythm
No fracture seen on pelvic X-ray

Progress

Clive was diagnosed with a suspected urinary tract infection (UTI) and started on oral antibiotics. He was seen by the physiotherapy team and found to be at his usual level of mobility. He was discharged home.

Is this an example of comprehensive geriatric assessment?
Is the diagnosis likely to be correct?
Is he at risk of readmission?
What could have been done differently?

Geriatric Medicine—The Basics

Biological ageing causes an accumulation of defects in our cells over time. Examples include damage to DNA sequences and clumps of abnormal proteins, such as amyloid (see Figure 1.1). Reduced flexibility of tissues, such as the lungs and blood vessels, develops due to loss of stretchy elastin protein and a build-up of fibrous collagen protein and calcium deposits. Molecular damage accumulation eventually leads to loss of cells, such as neurons, by apoptosis. The rate of this build-up varies between individuals, which is why chronological age is not a reliable determinant of function or resilience. The difference is partly explained by internal factors, like our genes, but also by external factors, such as smoking, sunlight exposure, diet, exercise, and accidents. Greater social deprivation is also associated with accelerated biological ageing. When enough cellular deficits have developed, then our organs work inefficiently. Ultimately, bodily function, both physical and cognitive, becomes impaired.

Most people accumulate long-term conditions over their lifespan. These are illnesses that can be managed with medicines but are usually incurable. Common examples include hypertension, chronic obstructive pulmonary disease (COPD), type 2 diabetes, and dementia. Multi-morbidity is a term for having more than one long-term condition. Clinical guidelines

Biological ageing

Accummulated cellular damage
DNA
Abnormal proteins

Reduced tissue elasticity
Increased collagen, reduced elastin, calcium deposition

Cell loss (apoptosis) triggered by accummulated cellular damage

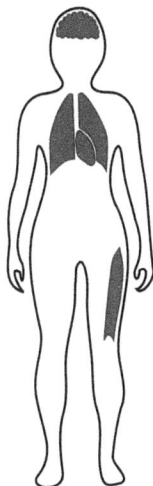

Organ effects

Brain - atrophy, small vessel ischaemic disease, amyloid deposition

Heart / lungs - loss of elasticity, increased pulse pressure, reduced heart diastolic relaxation, increased lung residual volume

Muscle - reduced muscle mass and strength (sarcopenia)

Figure 1.1 The effect of biological ageing on our body.

for the management of each condition promote prescribing. Consequently, multi-morbidity leads to polypharmacy. For people aged 85 and over in the UK, around 85% have multi-morbidity,[1] and around 25% take eight or more different medications each week.[2] A complex association exists between biological ageing, multi-morbidity, and polypharmacy. Each one is likely to promote the other two.

Frailty

Frailty is a recognisable state of vulnerability due to advanced biological ageing. For affected people, what appear to be 'minor' stressors can have a dramatic functional impact. People with frailty tend to present 'atypically' with illnesses, often with acute physical (i.e. falls or reduced mobility) and/or cognitive (i.e. delirium) decline. This is atypical to the presentations described in traditional medical textbooks but entirely typical for the most frequent users of modern healthcare. The recovery of people with frailty is slower and often incomplete compared to less frail people experiencing similar illnesses. People with frailty are more likely to experience adverse effects from medications, complications during hospitalisations, and more likely to die. Being armed with this knowledge can help tailor care to better suit their needs and personal goals. When frailty is unrecognised, the patient risks not getting the right help. Inappropriate and unhelpful terms like 'social admission' or 'acopia' may be attached. People with frailty often present with several problems at once, and these frequently include medication adverse effects.

Biological ageing is hard to assess at the bedside, as a result, there is no universally accepted and practical way to define frailty in clinical settings. Frailty should be seen as a continuum—people can have degrees of frailty. A commonly used assessment is the Clinical Frailty Scale (CFS) (see Table 1.1, focussed on categories 4 to 8 that we are most interested in).[3] More severe frailty is associated with greater functional impairment. Consequently, the

Table 1.1 A Summary of the Clinical Frailty Scale

Score	Frailty rating	Description
1–3	Non-frail	—
4	At risk	'Slowing down', less able to do strenuous activities, more sedentary
5	Mild	Affecting ability to do finances, use transport, may affect ability to go to shops/outdoors alone
6	Moderate	Require assistance with some personal care (e.g. bathing, supervision for dressing) and may struggle with stairs
7	Severe	Dependent on others for most/all aspects of personal care
8	Very severe	Completely dependent (i.e. mobility, personal care, feeding), close to the end of life
9	N/A	Receiving palliative care but not otherwise frail

degree of dependence on others is a useful surrogate marker. The functional impairment may be caused by physical and/or cognitive deficits.

Tips for Using the CFS

It is designed for people aged over 65, so not usually applicable to younger people. At times of acute illness, assessments should be based on function two weeks prior to becoming unwell. It should supplement, not replace, CGA (i.e. you still need to do an assessment). Accuracy may be improved by obtaining collateral history to verify abilities. Change in function is key—i.e. if they have never done their own finances, then this cannot be used as an indication of developing frailty.

Estimating degree of frailty contributes to patient care. It is not used to deny access to treatments but instead to inform choices. People with moderate to severe frailty are more likely to experience adverse effects with medicines or operations and are more likely to develop functional decline or die because of their illnesses. Effective shared decision-making requires optimising information for the individual patient. Recognising someone's pre-existing frailty also helps with diagnosing the cause of the most recent deterioration. A person with severe frailty who has dramatically changed in function may have only a minor change in health status, such as a new drug prescription or developed constipation, whereas a more robust person would need a larger insult to cause the same deficit. This can reduce the confusion brought about when we read that 'anything can cause delirium'.

Caring for People with Frailty

Good care is proactive. Potential problems are detected and prevented before they occur. Unwell people with frailty are less likely to be able to meet their own basic needs (e.g. nutrition, hydration, and toileting) and so it falls to us to anticipate these needs on top of their 'medical needs' to avoid deterioration. Ensure the person has a drink and call buzzer in easy reach when you leave their bedside. Put anything you moved away from the patient back to where it was. There is evidence that some aspects of frailty are reversible, for example, weight training to reverse sarcopenia. Such modification may not be achievable during an acute illness or admission. Focussing on preventing deterioration is key. The early promotion of mobility and steps to reduce the risk of delirium are core components of high-quality care. We will discuss these topics in later cases.

Care should be patient-centred with excellent communication. Ask patients what is important to them. What are their goals? Take opportunities to speak to relatives, with patient consent, and explore their ideas, concerns, and expectations, e.g. baseline function, current social difficulties, and discussions around treatment escalation plans. Patient respect and dignity must be preserved.

Involve the family or carers as often as possible if the person is happy for this to happen. Frail older people are often only able to live independently with support and so, understanding the strain this is putting on loved ones is a crucial aspect of caring for your patient. Many cognitively impaired older people will benefit from the support of the people close to them in complex decision-making and also in enduring time away from home. In the UK, John's Campaign advocates for the ability of carers to be present at any time to support people with dementia while in hospital. This can be as simple as encouraging eating and as complex as staying with them throughout their physiotherapy assessment and overnight if distressed. Car parking permits and free meals in the hospital canteen are important additions to show carers that their input is valuable.

Comprehensive Geriatric Assessment

Comprehensive geriatric assessment (CGA) is the way to evaluate medical complexity. It is an evidence-based intervention, leading to a greater chance of being alive and in one's own home a year later.[4] It has similarities with a standard medical assessment but with extra elements. The core components are shown in Table 1.2. Additional domains and assessments will sometimes be required, such as speech and language therapy. Collateral history is likely to be required to get the optimal information. This also represents a chance to clarify aspects of usual function and identify carer stress. It is a multi-disciplinary team assessment usually

Table 1.2 The Core Components of CGA

Medical	History, including medications, physical examination Avoid unhelpful terms like 'poor historian'—you are the historian, if necessary, ask elsewhere, e.g. the relatives, carers, or usual doctor
Psychological	Cognition and mood
Social	Care—current provision or support Environment—property type, other occupants, stairs, equipment Alcohol/smoking —risk of withdrawal, nicotine replacement therapy?
Functional	Mobility/ability to do self-care

performed by several people in collaboration. The outcome is likely to be the identification of multiple problems. Assessment alone is not very helpful. The key step is formulating a problem list and management plan. Tackle the most important and/or reversible issues first.

Diagnosing UTI

UTI is commonly overdiagnosed in older people. The result is that the real problem isn't identified, so the patient can't get better, and there is unnecessary exposure to antibiotics. It is reasonable to suspect a UTI in someone with an acute onset of urinary symptoms, such as dysuria and increased urinary frequency. But these do not always indicate a UTI and are not reported by everyone with a UTI, for example, people with a urinary catheter, delirium, or dementia. Urinary symptoms that have been present for more than a week are very unlikely to be caused by a UTI. People prescribed sodium-glucose co-transporter 2 inhibitors (e.g. dapagliflozin) are at increased risk of developing a UTI.

There are no reliable clinical signs for UTI. Suprapubic tenderness is not caused by bacteria in the urine. It can be a sign of urinary retention, and a bladder scan could help rule this out. In older men, one or both of an enlarged prostate gland and constipation are common causes of urinary retention. Smelling of urine is not a sign of UTI. It is a sign of urinary incontinence and/or reduced ability to maintain personal hygiene. This may happen to anyone in the context of an acute illness. Urine being strong-smelling, dark-coloured, or cloudy is also not a reliable sign of UTI but may indicate dehydration. Asymptomatic bacteriuria is the finding of bacteria in the urine without attributable symptoms. It is common, affecting 25–50% of older people with frailty in hospitals and everyone with a long-term catheter. This means that urinalysis (i.e. dipstick leucocytes and nitrites) and urine culture cannot be used to diagnose UTI in our population.

So, how can we diagnose UTI? It is best to only diagnose UTI when at least two of the following three criteria are met:

- Acute onset urinary symptoms (e.g. dysuria, frequency or urgency)
- Signs of an infection (i.e. pyrexia, raised serum white blood cell count or high C-reactive protein (e.g. > 50 mg/L))
- There is no better alternative explanation for symptoms and signs

In other situations, search for an alternative explanation for your patient's presentation. When a diagnosis of UTI is made, send a urine sample to the laboratory and prescribe empirical antibiotics according to your hospital guidelines while you await sensitivities based on culture. Patients with a urinary catheter should have it changed at the start of UTI treatment to maximise the chance of successful resolution. 'Recurrent UTI' may simply describe repeated episodes of functional decline or delirium. It should prompt a review of previous test results and consideration of alternative diagnoses. If often indicates progressive frailty or cognitive decline where CGA would be of value, not a urological problem.

What about Clive?

The assessment that Clive received in the emergency department followed a logical process and wasn't inherently wrong, but it didn't get to the bottom of his problems. It is very unlikely that he had a UTI and so the actual issues persist, and he is likely to be readmitted soon (N.B. his C-reactive protein is marginally elevated above the reference value but not high enough to suggest a significant inflammatory process).

Clive is mildly frail (CFS 5) and needs some help from his son for usual daily activities. He presents with a fall, which has many possible causes, which we will discuss in later cases. When we look at his medical history, there are already a few things to think about. Taking medications for hypertension is associated with a risk of orthostatic hypotension. This could have caused a transient drop in blood pressure when he got out of bed, which can occur without feeling light-headed. Osteoarthritis could impair his gait and balance. His type 2 diabetes is tightly controlled (Hb_{A1C} 43). Hypoglycaemia could have contributed to his fall, and a reduction in his glucose-lowering medication may be appropriate. Cognitive impairment also increases the risk of falling. For example, he might forget to move more cautiously now that his balance is less good.

Clive smells of urine because he fell over and couldn't get to the toilet. This has made him feel embarrassed. He needs assistance right away to get washed and put on clean clothes to restore his dignity. When asked, he said that his main priorities in life are maintaining his independence and spending time with his family. We can use this information when discussing the risks and benefits of his medications to help achieve his goals. We should perform a cognitive assessment and, with his permission, get some collateral history from his son. We should measure his lying and standing blood pressure to detect any deficit. A bladder scan can rule out urinary retention. In addition to the physiotherapy assessment, an occupational therapy assessment can detect beneficial adaptations, such as a second banister rail on his stairs. It may be possible to improve his toilet access, which could include a bedside commode or urine bottle for overnight. There's more we could do but that's enough to get us started. Through the following cases, we will build on these concepts.

Key Points

- UTI is frequently overdiagnosed.
- CGA is how we assess older people with medical complexity.
- Assessing frailty can help personalise care.
- People with frailty often present with several problems at once, and these frequently include medication adverse effects.
- People with moderate to severe frailty are more likely to experience adverse effects with medicines or operations and are more likely to develop functional decline or die because of their illnesses.
- The foundations of high-quality care include patient respect and dignity. If you fail to achieve this, then no amount of medical knowledge can resurrect the care that you deliver.

Further Reading

1. *Chief Medical Officer's Annual Report 2023*. Health in an Ageing Society.
2. *Health Survey for England 2016*. digital.nhs.uk

3. Rockwood K, Song X, MacKnight C, et al. A global clinical measure of fitness and frailty in elderly people. *CMAJ* 2005;173:489–95. https://doi.org/10.1503/cmaj.050051

4. Ellis G, Gardner M, Tsiachristas A, et al. Comprehensive geriatric assessment for older adults admitted to hospital. *Cochrane Database Syst Rev* 2017;Issue 9. Art. No.: CD006211. https://doi.org/10.1002/14651858.CD006211.pub3

Case 2

Geeta

Geeta is an 81-year-old retired nurse. The paramedics who brought her into hospital handed over that she had been well the previous night, but at 8 AM, her carer thought she wasn't her usual self. Geeta's speech appeared slurred. When the carer returned at 11 AM, she looked worse, she hadn't eaten any of the breakfast that had been prepared for her, and the right side of her face was drooping. Geeta didn't report any symptoms when asked.

Past Medical History

Dementia—diagnosed two years ago and labelled as mixed aetiology
Parkinson's disease—diagnosed 12 years ago
Poor hearing
Left shoulder surgery

Medication

Aspirin 75 mg od	Co-careldopa 125 mg qds (8 AM, 11 AM, 2 PM, 5 PM)
Colecalciferol 800 units od	Cyanocobalamin 50 mcg od
Levothyroxine 25 mcg od	Memantine 20 mg od

Social History

Geeta lives in sheltered accommodation with two carers attending four times a day. She needs help to mobilise using a transfer aid and the assistance of two people. The carers assist Geeta with her medications, washing, dressing, and meals. She has dual incontinence that is managed with pads. She has limited awareness of the need to go to the toilet. Her carer reported that although her short-term memory was poor, she would usually communicate in full sentences and is able to express her needs. She does not smoke or drink alcohol.

Examination

Geeta was lying on a bed, leaning to the left. She appeared comfortable. She was able to follow one-stage but not two-stage commands. There was no facial asymmetry at that time. Her eyes were not deviated to one side. She could not follow the instructions for visual field

DOI: 10.1201/9781003582007-2

examination but blinked to confrontation stimulus on either side. Initially, she looked a little dyskinetic, but this settled during the examination. There was no pronator drift, and her power was not reduced in any limb. There was mild generalised increased tone. Cognitive impairment was present, she had limited speech and gave one-word answers to most questions, but expressive dysphasia was not detected.

Six-Item Screener 0/6

BP 122/80 mmHg, pulse 70 bpm, 97% air, temperature 35.9°C, respiratory rate 20/min

Investigations

Biochemistry	Value	Reference range	Haematology	Value	Reference range
Sodium	152	133–146 mmol/L	Haemoglobin	138	115–165 g/L
Potassium	3.4	3.5–5.3 mmol/L	MCV	98	82–100 fL
Urea	17.6	2.5–7.8 mmol/L	White cell count	9.4	4–11 10^9/L
Creatinine	71	49–90 umol/L	Platelets	61	140–400 10^9/L
C-reactive protein	94	< 5 mg/L			
Albumin	29	35–50 g/L	Vitamin B_{12}	247	150–1000 ng/L
TSH	2.1	0.3–4.5 mIU/L			

Urea 4.9 and creatinine 64 when last tested a few months ago. Calcium and liver blood tests all within normal range. Vitamin B_{12} was 138 four years ago.

ECG—sinus rhythm, 68 bpm, no significant abnormality

Chest X-ray—no focal consolidation

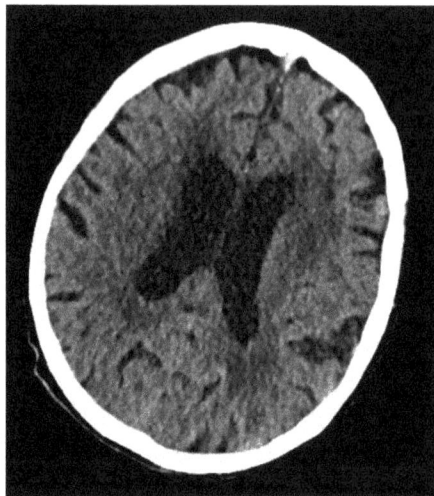

Figure 2.1 CT brain scan.

Progress

A bedside swallow test was performed, i.e. she was carefully observed after being offered a teaspoon of water, and a delayed swallow was noted. The speech and language therapy (SLT) team were asked to review her. With SLT, she was given a small amount of normal consistency fluids but then had a prolonged bout of coughing that took three minutes to subside. After this, the assessment was repeated. This time, there were no overt signs of aspiration. She needed prompting to take small sips. A level four pureed diet was also successfully trialled. The swallowing problem was described as moderate to severe oropharyngeal dysphagia, secondary to an acute decompensation on a background of dementia and parkinsonism. The SLT recommendations are that she is only offered food when upright and alert, small amounts slowly. Geeta could have normal consistency fluids via an open cup with a double-handed beaker (no straws or spouted beakers) and level four pureed diet taken from a teaspoon. She will need full support and supervision for any oral intake and will need prompting to eat and drink.

What can be seen on Geeta's CT brain scan?
Has she had a stroke?
What other reasons for her deterioration are likely?
What do her blood tests show?
Would you change her Parkinson's disease treatment?
Would you change any of her other medications?
What are the risks and benefits of thickened fluids?

Diagnosis of Stroke

An acute stroke, or transient ischaemic attack (TIA), causes a sudden onset of a focal neurological deficit. Clinical features are worst at the time of onset and tend to gradually improve over time. Deficits are described as 'negative' (e.g. weakness, visual loss, sensory loss) rather than 'positive' (e.g. twitching, flashing lights, 'pins and needles' sensation). Brain imaging can assist with diagnosis. CT scanning can easily detect acute intracerebral bleeding and may detect early changes of ischaemic stroke if the infarct is large. MRI scanning is more sensitive to detect early infarcts, especially if only small.

Geeta initially had slurred speech. This can be caused by a wide variety of problems, such as poorly fitting dentures or alcohol intoxication, and is not necessarily due to a focal brain lesion. Her symptoms gradually worsened over several hours. The assessment of facial drooping can be subjective. If leaning to one side, then gravity may alter facial appearance. Examination in hospital hadn't detected a focal neurological deficit. No acute lesion was seen on her brain CT scan (but this may not show a small stroke or detect early changes within the first few hours). Taking all of this into account, it is unlikely that acute stroke or TIA was the reason she became unwell.

Cause of Deterioration

Geeta has had an acute deterioration in her physical (e.g. didn't eat breakfast, leaning to left) and cognitive function (e.g. single-word answers). She scored poorly on the Six-Item Screener

Table 2.1 U PINCH ME Assessment for Geeta

*U*rine retention	This could be caused by constipation; Geeta takes memantine and is dehydrated, risk of absolute retention greater in men due to prostatic enlargement
*P*ain	Geeta is not complaining of pain (N.B. dementia may affect ability to express needs) and looks comfortable at rest
*I*nfection	C-reactive protein is raised but WCC normal, no obvious source of infection (incontinence is longstanding), is at risk of aspiration pneumonia, could have a viral illness
*N*utrition	No obvious change prior to onset but now in hospital, which could affect intake, vitamin B_{12} discussed later
*C*onstipation	Consider rectal examination, complete bowel chart, speak to carers for more information
*H*ydration	Blood tests suggest dehydration, i.e. high sodium and urea, Geeta's creatinine may not be raised due to sarcopenia
*M*edications	No known recent change, co-careldopa can affect cognition
*E*nvironment	No change prior to onset but may now be made worse through being in an unfamiliar hospital environment

brief cognitive test [see Case 3]. Given her degree of frailty, she is very vulnerable to any acute illness and likely to present with this type of non-specific decline. This is where the skills of geriatric medicine have great value. CGA is the solution. The medical term for this type of acute cognitive change is delirium, which has multiple possible causes. The mnemonic 'U PINCH ME' can be a helpful guide for detecting common precipitants (see Table 2.1).

Blood Test Results

A raised serum sodium is almost always due to dehydration but is not present in all people with dehydration. The marked rise in urea with a smaller rise in creatinine would also fit with this. Another possibility for the high urea is a gastrointestinal bleed, but nothing in her history suggests this, her Hb is in the normal range, and it wouldn't cause a high sodium. Rehydrating her will improve her sodium. We want to avoid over-rapid correction. When using intravenous fluids, a balanced solution like Hartmann's fluid is preferable to 5% glucose.

Geeta's serum C-reactive protein is elevated but this is non-specific, and there isn't an obvious cause. While possible to do a broad range of tests to rule out numerous pathologies, we might just treat the things we know about first and then repeat her blood tests afterwards. Her low albumin could be due to renal loss, reduced formation due to liver disease, or chronic inflammatory disease. Again, we could do a range of tests to look for an explanation, but this isn't always helpful. One of the skills of geriatric medicine is knowing when not to do all the things that we could do. Given Geeta's cognitive impairment, we can have a discussion with her and her next of kin to identify what is in Geeta's best interests.

A low platelet count can be caused by reduced formation due to bone marrow diseases (most likely myelodysplasia for Geeta, her vitamin B_{12} deficiency has been corrected), autoimmune disease, disseminated intravascular coagulation, infections, or medication adverse effects (e.g. quinine, sulpha-antibiotics, anticonvulsants). How low would Geeta's platelets have to get for us to stop her aspirin? Typical guidance suggests caution once below 50 but what is the risk/benefit for her? There is no secondary vascular prevention indication in her past medical history. Her platelet count may improve outside of this acute illness, so we could repeat the test once she has recovered. It is sensible that we would consider deprescribing the aspirin, and we could discuss this with her next of kin.

Parkinson's Disease Treatment

Parkinson's disease (PD) is an idiopathic neurodegenerative condition resulting in reduced intracerebral dopamine pathways. Motor symptoms include slowness, stiffness, resting tremor, and gait disturbance. Treatments for PD mainly help to control motor symptoms. Unfortunately, they do not have a disease-modifying role. Receipt of the correct medication at the correct time is vital to preserve physical function. Anti-dopamine medications must be avoided (e.g. antipsychotics and metoclopramide). Non-motor symptoms include cognitive impairment, constipation, sleep disturbance, urinary disorders, and swallow impairment. Proactive care seeks out such problems.

The 'Get It On Time' campaign in the UK highlights the challenges that people with PD have in hospital. Despite years of advocacy from voluntary organisations, and many quality improvement endeavours, there are very frequent delays in giving people their PD medicines. Incorporating support from family and carers, the use of alarms within electronic systems or nurses' devices, and patient-controlled medication processes can help.

At times of reduced oral intake or impaired swallowing (e.g. acute illness or peri-operatively), medication options include switching to a liquid form (i.e. co-beneldopa dispersible—which can be given down a nasogastric [NG] tube if necessary), rotigotine patches (a dopamine agonist), or a subcutaneous apomorphine infusion (specialist use only). There may be other options for people with swallow impairment who can only take food in a specific consistency. For example, standard release co-careldopa can be crushed and mixed with yogurt-consistency foods. Specialist advice should be sought as soon as possible. Conversion charts for PD drugs to equivalent doses of dispersible co-beneldopa are available online.

The main aim of giving some regular dopaminergic treatment with different delivery/formulation in this setting is to avoid the neuroleptic malignant-like syndrome from abrupt drug withdrawal. This is more common when people are routinely taking high doses of PD medication. The side effect profile of dopamine receptor agonists (e.g. rotigotine) is different from levodopa-based treatments with greater risk of neuropsychiatric symptoms, so it is a particularly difficult situation when someone with PD has delirium and swallowing problems. Agreed hospital policies and specialist advice access are important safety features for this scenario.

Motor symptoms become more complex in advanced PD and are harder to control. Medication doses have a shorter duration of action. People with PD develop wearing-off towards the end of doses and experience fluctuations between symptom control and undertreatment. Superimposed dyskinesia (choreoathetoid movements) also becomes more likely.

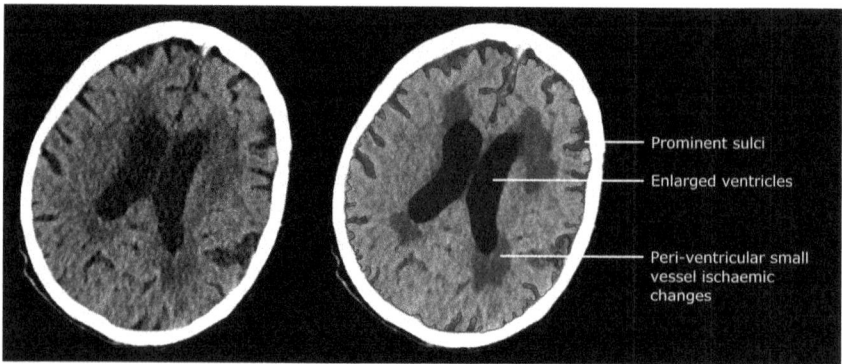

Prominent sulci

Enlarged ventricles

Peri-ventricular small vessel ischaemic changes

Figure 2.2 Abnormalities visible on Geeta's brain CT scan.

Although people with dementia and/or small vessel cerebrovascular disease can get parkinsonism, the diagnosis of PD is likely to be correct for Geeta. She was diagnosed over ten years ago and has been followed up in a specialist PD service since then. Clinic letters suggest she had a good symptomatic response to levodopa when it was first commenced. However, things change over time, and her brain CT scan now shows widespread atrophy and small vessel ischaemic lesions in addition to the non-visible underlying PD pathology (see Figure 2.2). This multi-morbidity could affect the risk-benefit balance of medications for PD. Geeta's associated cognitive impairment, reduced swallow, and dyskinesia all suggest that she is coming to the end-stage of PD. Identifying this can help with discussions around future wishes and advance care planning.

Other Medications

Reducing Geeta's medication burden could be helpful, especially given her current swallowing difficulty. As already discussed, it is worth considering whether the continued use of aspirin for primary vascular prevention is still in her best interests. It will not prevent the progression of cerebrovascular small vessel disease. She has been on a very low dose of levothyroxine for years. Looking through her past blood test results, her TSH has never been recorded above 10, which is classified as subclinical hypothyroidism. Evidence does not suggest a benefit from treatment. We could discuss deprescribing, possibly with a repeat TSH in a couple of months' time to be sure of no adverse effect. Cyanocobalamin is an oral replacement for vitamin B_{12}. Once replete, bodily vitamin B_{12} stores can last for more than a year. Options for Geeta include leaving this alone, stopping the cyanocobalamin tablet, and repeating vitamin B_{12} measurement in three months' time or switching to a three-monthly intramuscular injection if she struggles to swallow a tablet. Colecalciferol is discussed more in later cases. Deprescribing this can also be considered.

Risk-Benefit of Thickened Fluids

Thickened fluids are sometimes recommended for people with an impaired swallow mechanism. In theory, thickened fluids move more slowly through the mouth, which allows more time to direct them down the oesophagus and away from one's airway. A key disadvantage is that people tend not to like the altered consistency and taste. This could lead to avoiding fluids and risking dehydration. There is only weak scientific evidence that thickened fluids improve outcomes.[1] This doesn't mean that a trial of thickened fluids is wrong but does underline the need for their consideration on an individual basis. Work with the SLT team in the best interests of the patient. Other adjustments may work better for them.

A modified diet may be recommended for people with dysphagia. A standardised grading of food consistency has been described.[2] Level zero liquids include normal water. Level seven foods are the most solid and include things like steak. Going from zero to seven, substances increase in viscosity. The distinction between food and drink becomes blurred around level three to four with pureed or yogurt-like consistencies.

A plan to keep an older person with frailty 'nil by mouth' in hospital is rarely helpful. Whatever the cause, if they cannot swallow, it is a very serious situation that we need to recognise, discuss, and think about the benefits and risks of the decisions made. If the person is not allowed to eat or drink at all, it will certainly rapidly cause trouble in terms of energy, bowels and bladder function, and mobility and will accelerate deconditioning. It is also distressing for cognitively impaired people to be kept from eating and drinking without understanding why. What is the real risk we are mitigating? Is it the potential to aspirate or distressing symptoms of coughing/choking? 'Free water protocol' involves good mouth care and normal water to drink; it doesn't appear to increase the risk of aspiration pneumonia but may improve fluid intake, even in very difficult situations.[3] Sometimes a palliative approach is appropriate. 'Risk feeding' is a term for accepting the intake of an appropriately modified diet, for patient comfort, even though there is a high probability of aspiration.

NG feeding tube placement is a possible short-term fix for a swallowing problem but can be uncomfortable and is often poorly tolerated. NG feeding for people who have lost the ability to swallow due to dementia has not been shown to improve survival or quality of life and may lead to complications, including pressure ulcers.[4] NG feeding in people with delirium is very difficult and risky, sometimes leading to physical or chemical restraint, which is counterproductive in terms of managing their delirium. It has been used for people with PD who are acutely unwell to give them levodopa and maintain nutrition, but its practical challenges are many and an individualised assessment is crucial.

What about Geeta?

Geeta has severe frailty (CFS 7) and came into hospital because of an acute deterioration in her health. Treatment of a causative illness and appropriate rehabilitation may lead to recovery. Although, so far, we haven't diagnosed or treated anything. Her function is likely to deteriorate over time due to the already known conditions. This is a frequent dilemma in geriatric medicine: We want to give her the best chance of recovery but also don't want to keep her in hospital if not helpful.

Because of swallowing problems, Geeta is likely to need extra assistance eating and drinking in the future. The duration of the calls by her carers may need to increase to allow for this. Despite care four times a day, there will be long periods when she is alone at home, including overnight. While she is in hospital, the ward team can keep an eye on her overnight needs. Does your patient get up out of bed? If they need the toilet, can they get themselves there and back without assistance? Because Geeta has limited awareness of the need to go and wears containment pads, this may not be an issue for her. But these are important factors to determine whether she could return to sheltered accommodation or if 24-hour support, as provided in a care home, needs to be considered.

Geeta needs help with all her personal care. She has a very high risk of future deterioration, including aspiration pneumonia. She is likely to be in the last year of her life. If not already done, advance care planning should be initiated during her current hospital admission.

Key Points

- Acute stroke causes a sudden onset of a focal neurological deficit.
- People with frailty are very vulnerable to any acute illness and likely to present with non-specific functional or cognitive decline.
- Delirium can be caused by any acute illness and numerous medications.
- For people with PD, receipt of the correct medication at the correct time is vital to preserve physical function.
- Thickened fluids can help some people with swallow problems, but with a balance of risks and benefits, choices need to be individualised.

Further Reading

1. O'Keeffe ST. Use of modified diets to prevent aspiration in oropharyngeal dysphagia: is current practice justified? *BMC Geriatr* 2018;18:167. https://doi.org/10.1186/s12877-018-0839-7

2. *The International Dysphagia Diet Standardisation Initiative*. https://www.iddsi.org/standards/framework

3. Gaidos S, Hrdlicka HC, Corbett J. Implementation of a free water protocol at a long term acute care hospital. *Sci Rep* 2023;13:2626. https://doi.org/10.1038/s41598-023-29448-5

4. Davies N, Barrado-Martín Y, Vickerstaff V, et al. Enteral tube feeding for people with severe dementia. *Cochrane Database Syst Rev* 2021;Issue 8. Art. No.: CD013503. https://doi.org/10.1002/14651858.CD013503.pub2

Case 3

Margaret

Margaret is a 77-year-old woman whose memory has gradually declined. She was diagnosed with mild cognitive impairment seven years ago and then Alzheimer's dementia five years ago. She is known to the local community psychiatry team who have visited her at home many times. She has had several months of delusional symptoms and confabulated stories, which have gradually escalated. Over the last few weeks, she had become more paranoid, believing that her neighbour was trying to kill her and her cat.

Margaret's granddaughter became very worried after an incident where Margaret was brought home by the police after being found wandering outdoors at 3 AM in her dressing gown. She had initially refused to go home because of fear about her neighbour. Her granddaughter had stayed with her that night. With unfortunate timing, her son happened to be on holiday for a week at the time. In the morning, a phone call was made to social services to see if an emergency respite placement could be arranged. The duty social worker requested a medical review to see if the change in her behaviour was due to an acute illness. Her GP was already concerned and had sent a urine sample several days ago, which grew *E. coli*, but Margaret was no better after the two days of antibiotics administered so far, which her granddaughter had supervised her taking.

Later that day, one of Margaret's neighbours reported that she knocked on his door then entered the house as soon as he opened it. She was frantic and distressed, stating there was someone in her house and a different neighbour had killed her cat. Her granddaughter knew that things couldn't go on like this. An ambulance was called, and she was brought to hospital.

When asked, Margaret did not know why she was in hospital. She did not have any pain, urine, bowel, or chest symptoms and did not describe any current delusions or hallucinations. Her son cut his holiday short and came to the hospital to see his mother. Two months prior to this admission, he had become concerned when Margaret was having difficulty taking her medication as prescribed and had sometimes taken several day's medication over a 24-hour period. Her son was also worried that she was leaving her front door open.

Past Medical History

Alzheimer's dementia—diagnosed five years ago
Hypertension
Vitamin B_{12} deficiency

DOI: 10.1201/9781003582007-3

Medication

Atorvastatin 40 mg od	Citalopram 20 mg od
Donepezil 10 mg od	Losartan 100 mg od
Memantine 20 mg od	Paracetamol 1 g bd
Vitamin B$_{12}$ intramuscular injections three-monthly	Nitrofurantoin 100 mg MR bd for three days started two days ago

Social History

Margaret lives alone except for her 12-year-old cat, called Milly. She is usually independent with self-care. Her granddaughter does her shopping and buys ready meals, which Margaret can heat up in her microwave. She has a care package in place twice a day for medication prompts. Her son visits for an hour each evening when he finishes work and again on Saturday and Sunday mornings. He has Lasting Power of Attorney for her financial affairs. She has never smoked and only occasionally drinks alcohol. She has not driven a car for over seven years.

Examination

Margaret was sitting in a chair and had a normal level of alertness. She had normal tone in all limbs and no focal weakness. She had a soft systolic heart murmur. Her chest was clear, and there was no peripheral oedema. Abdomen soft and non-tender. She independently mobilised to the toilet in the emergency department.

Six-Item Screener 1/6

4AT 7/12

BP 168/87, pulse 103 bpm, respiratory rate 19/min, oxygen saturation 96% air, temperature 36.4°C

Investigations

Biochemistry	Value	Reference range	Haematology	Value	Reference range
Sodium	140	133–146 mmol/L	Haemoglobin	125	115–165 g/L
Potassium	3.6	3.5–5.3 mmol/L	MCV	84	82–100 fL
Urea	2.6	2.5–7.8 mmol/L	White cell count	6.3	4–11 10⁹/L
Creatinine	55	49–90 umol/L	Platelets	303	140–400 10⁹/L
C-reactive protein	1	< 5 mg/L			
Adjusted calcium	2.21	2.2–2.6 mmol/L			

Viral swab for influenza/COVID was negative.
Liver function blood tests were all normal.
Urine culture, taken three days ago, grew *E. coli* sensitive to all antibiotics.

Does Margaret have a urinary tract infection?
What is the cause of the deterioration in her cognition?

Diagnosing Urinary Tract Infection

Diagnosing UTI was also discussed in Case 1. Margaret hasn't reported any urinary tract symptoms, but this could have been affected by dementia. She doesn't have any clinical evidence of an infection—i.e. WCC, C-reactive protein, and temperature are all within the normal range. Her symptoms have fluctuated a bit but have been present for several months. Her GP had sent a urine culture prior to admission, which grew *E. coli*. However, the high prevalence of asymptomatic bacteriuria in older people with frailty means that urine culture cannot be used to diagnose UTI, but it could help with choosing the most suitable antibiotic after a diagnosis has been made. Margaret didn't get any better after receiving antibiotics in the community, but she had only started them recently. On balance, it is very unlikely that her symptoms are due to a UTI.

Cognitive Impairment

Delirium and dementia cause cognitive impairment. It can also sometimes be mimicked by severe depression. Cognitive impairment cannot be reliably detected if not specifically tested for. In acute medical settings, it is often missed for this reason. This can have a great impact on effective shared decision-making, consent to treatment, and discharge planning. Simple bedside tests include the Six-Item Screener (see later) and asking the patient to list the months of the year in reverse order (a test of attention, which is impaired in delirium). Longer tests can help define the specific aspects of cognition that are affected and rate severity. These include the Montreal Cognitive Assessment (MOCA), scored out of 30, and the Addenbrooke's Cognitive Examination version 3 (ACE-III), scored out of 100. With both tests, lower scores represent more severe cognitive decline. Looking through the clinical records for prior scores can help define progression.

Six-Item Screener

Give the patient three items to remember, ask them to repeat the items to ensure that have heard correctly—e.g. key, lemon, and table

Ask the patient the current day of the week [1 point]
Ask the patient the current month [1 point]
Ask the patient the current year [1 point]
Then ask the patient to repeat the three items from earlier [1 point for each correct]
Total score 0 to 6. A score of 4 or less suggests that further assessment may be required.

Once cognitive impairment has been identified, a collateral history from someone who knows the patient is the most helpful next step. Sometimes, relatives overestimate their loved one's prior abilities (perhaps because we don't tend to specifically look for problems—we see what we want to see). Useful questions can be based around function. For example, does the patient still drive, use the telephone, recognise familiar faces, and manage their finances, and could they get the bus into town by themselves? One potential difficulty is that the severity of cognitive deficits can fluctuate. This is characteristic of delirium but can occur in people with dementia, who may function worse in the evenings, a phenomenon called 'sundowning'. In hospitals, the patient may appear fine during the daytime ward round but cause pandemonium overnight.

Delirium

Delirium is an acute confusional state characterised by recent onset, fluctuations in severity, and reduced attention. It can be caused by any illness in a vulnerable person. Someone with delirium may be hyperactive or hypoactive to varying degrees. Hyperactivity can range from being fidgety and picking at bedclothes to pacing around and aggression. Hypoactivity can range from mild drowsiness, which is easily overlooked, to unconsciousness. Affected people can cycle between these states of alertness. At times, there may be associated delusions and hallucinations. In older people with frailty, delirium can be slow to improve and may not fully resolve. Some degree of persisting impairment is likely at the time of discharge. People tend to function optimally in their own homes, and recovery can still occur once away from the bustle of acute hospital wards.

The key features of delirium are altered alertness, cognitive deficit, reduced attention, and acute onset and/or fluctuating severity. The 4AT is a helpful assessment tool for delirium because it targets these four aspects.[1] The 4AT is scored from 0 to 12. A score of 0 makes delirium unlikely, whereas a score of 4 or more makes delirium likely.

Dementia

Dementia is a chronic progressive impairment of cognitive function. Numerous pathological processes can contribute. Dementia is often classified according to the most likely underlying pathology. In older people with frailty, this can be misleading. Most will have a combination of several neurodegenerative processes and vascular lesions affecting their brain function. The commonest diagnoses are Alzheimer's disease (a form of neurodegeneration) and vascular dementia.

Dementia commonly affects memory but not always. Predominantly, frontal lobe pathology affects personality, the ability to make judgments, and performing complex tasks. This pattern can be seen with vascular dementia or frontotemporal dementia. Dementia with Lewy bodies (DLB) is another relatively common form. DLB usually presents with a combination of cognitive impairment and parkinsonism. The cognitive impairment may resemble delirium with altered alertness and fluctuating severity and is sometimes associated with delusions/hallucinations. People with DLB are very sensitive to antipsychotic drugs, and so these must be avoided.

People with dementia can develop challenging behaviours. The term 'behavioural and psychological symptoms of dementia' (BPSD) is sometimes attached. Examples include wandering, sleep disturbance, repetitive questioning, psychosis, aggression, and socially inappropriate behaviours. BPSD can spontaneously appear and disappear. Possible triggers include hospital admission.

Delirium and Dementia

People with dementia are very prone to delirium, and this can be hard to distinguish from BPSD. Illnesses and environmental changes (e.g. hospital admission) easily trigger increased confusion. It is best to assume some degree of delirium in everyone with cognitive impairment until proven otherwise.

Table 3.1 Common Medications that Can Impair Cognition

Medication type	Examples
Anticholinergics	Solifenacin, amitriptyline, many medications have some anticholinergic properties [see Case 9]
Sedatives	Diazepam, zopiclone
Antipsychotics	Quetiapine, risperidone
Opiates	Codeine, morphine, oxycodone

Managing acute cognitive decline

Thorough assessment should look for, and mitigate, potential triggers, such as acute illnesses. The mnemonic 'U PINCH ME' can help this process, as discussed in Case 2. Pain can present differently in people with dementia who can find it hard to express themselves. Tools such as the Abbey Pain Scale or PAIN-AD can help. Medications that impair cognition should be identified (see Table 3.1). If possible, they should be withheld temporarily, stopped permanently, or have their dose reduced. But caution is needed for medications with potential withdrawal adverse effects, such as benzodiazepines. Medical interventions should be minimised. For example, urinary catheterisation should be avoided unless necessary (e.g. urinary retention) and removed as soon as possible. A non-pharmacological approach is best for managing challenging behaviours.

Person-Centred Care

Person-centred care describes an approach for people with cognitive impairment that recognises them as an individual rather than a disease label. It involves getting to know more about them, enabling them to participate, and trying to see things from their perspective.[2] This can be assisted by getting a collateral history. Relatives or friends can also be asked to complete a 'This is me' document.[3]

When confronted with a challenging behaviour, start by having a conversation in a non-threatening manner. Position yourself at their eye level. Speak calmly, do not invade their personal space, and do not argue. Communication technique adaptations can help.[4] People with dementia experience the world differently to you and can find it difficult to express their needs. Try to understand the message rather than the words. Challenging behaviours can represent unmet needs. Is the person in pain, hungry, thirsty, or bored? Try offering things like food, drink, going for a walk, or using the toilet. Trying to steer the conversation away from the issue causing conflict may help. The presence of family members is likely to calm things down. Ask if they can come in. In times of crisis, postpone things that aren't immediately vital, such as CT head scanning or rectal examination. Behaviours are likely to fluctuate and improve over time.

Pharmacological Management

Antipsychotic and sedative medications can only be considered as a last resort for severe problems, like aggression, when all other options have been tried. Guidelines typically suggest a low dose of an antipsychotic or benzodiazepine. These medications may make confusion worse. They suppress brain function, which is the opposite of person-centred care. Hyperactive delirium may simply be converted into hypoactive delirium and recovery delayed. They have numerous potential adverse effects, including aspiration pneumonia, and falls. People with severe behavioural disturbance are likely to decline taking oral medications. The intramuscular route is sometimes used. This is likely to require several people to restrain the patient, which will probably worsen their agitation. These medications do not have an instantaneous onset of action like you see in the movies. It takes two hours for maximal effect to occur.[5]

What about Margaret?

Initial assessments have not found a reversible cause for Margaret's cognitive decline. Her son being away could have had some impact, but given the longer duration, it is not the key issue. We have not diagnosed an acute illness or found an obvious culprit medication. Her pulse and BP are mildly elevated, consistent with being in a state of distress. It is likely that her dementia has become more severe, with super-imposed BPSD. She does not need an admission to a hospital medical bed, and this could have a net negative impact on her cognitive state. Could she go home with the support of her family and community psychiatry input?

Margaret's family are doing a great job of supporting her living independently, but it is increasingly difficult, and her safety may now be at risk. Despite twice daily care and regular visits from her family, there are long periods of the day, over 20 hours, where she is alone at home. An increase in her care would reduce this time alone only a little bit. Wandering outdoors and leaving her front door open suggest that she now requires 24-hour supervision. It is unrealistic to think that her granddaughter could stay over every night in the future. This would be incredibly demanding of her time and energy. Moving to sheltered accommodation or 24-hour care in a residential home that specialises in dementia care are options to consider with her and her family. She may not be able to take her cat, Milly, with her. Would someone else be able to look after Milly? Her son reported that she took all her medications at once recently. Although a carer already assists with medication-taking, her tablets need to be locked away between administration times. We should also consider if they are all still beneficial. Is taking atorvastatin and losartan for vascular prevention still an important goal given her cognitive impairment? Antidepressants have been shown to be less effective in people with dementia, and citalopram could also be considered for withdrawal.

An assessment of Margaret's mental capacity to decide her place of residence may be needed (see Case 6). If she lacks capacity, a decision will be made in her best interests. It should balance restriction of liberty and safety, while trying to respect her values and wishes. An emergency respite placement in a care home that specialises in dementia care is an option that may allow time to consider the right steps going forward. Her condition might improve. In the short term, moving to a new and unfamiliar residence is likely to affect her function, such as oral intake and falls risk. An antipsychotic medication could be tried to reduce her delusions, but there must be a balance of risks and potential benefits. BPSD symptoms may diminish with time and in a stable environment. If medication is started, the lowest effective dose should be used for the shortest period. Regular review and consideration of deprescribing would be necessary.

Although Margaret is not physically impaired, she has cognitive frailty. An ACE-III less than 82 is consistent with dementia. Her score was 71 six months ago. Although her condition is fluctuating, two weeks ago, she had moderate to severe dementia, giving her CFS 6 or 7. She is at high risk of deterioration, and this is an opportunity for advance care planning. In the future, would she want to come back to hospital for treatment of a severe medical illness or prefer to have palliative care in the community?

Key Points

- Be careful not to overdiagnose UTI.
- Cognitive impairment cannot be reliably detected if not specifically tested for, so make it make it part of your routine practice.
- Use a person-centred approach to manage people with challenging behaviours.

Further Reading

1. www.the4at.com
2. www.alzheimers.org.uk/about-dementia/treatments/person-centred-care
3. www.alzheimers.org.uk/get-support/publications-factsheets/this-is-me
4. www.alzheimers.org.uk/about-dementia/symptoms-and-diagnosis/symptoms/how-to-communicate-dementia
5. Meehan KM, Wang H, David SR, et al. Comparison of rapidly acting intramuscular olanzapine, lorazepam, and placebo: a double-blind, randomized study in acutely agitated patients with dementia. *Neuropsychopharmacology* 2002;26:494–504. https://doi.org/10.1016/S0893–133X(01)00365–7

Case 4

Joan

Joan is a 92-year-old retired estate agent who presented to hospital following an unwitnessed fall. She had been found by her daughter on the floor next to their sofa. Her condition had been declining over the last few weeks. She had had multiple falls. A number of these occurred when getting out of bed overnight, and consequently, she now sleeps on the sofa downstairs. Her mobility and oral intake had declined. She did not report any pain. She had no current chest, urine, or bowel symptoms.

Past Medical History

Hypertension
Stroke—partial anterior cerebral circulation infarction 12 years ago
Chronic cognitive impairment (no dementia diagnosis)
Epilepsy—no seizures for over 30 years
Falls
Fractured right neck of femur six years ago

Medication

Alendronate 70 mg weekly (since hip fracture)	Atorvastatin 20 mg od (since stroke)
Calcium and vitamin D one tablet twice daily	Clopidogrel 75 mg once daily
Lercanidipine 10 mg once daily	Phenytoin sodium 200 mg once daily

Social History

Joan lives with her daughter in a house. They have two cats. Due to declining mobility, she now needs a great deal of assistance, such as accessing the toilet. Her daughter sometimes carries her there. Joan and her daughter both feel the current home set-up is working but worry about frequent falls. She is an ex-smoker, having stopped over 50 years ago.

Examination

Joan has low muscle mass. There were bilateral periorbital bruises and further bruising on her cheeks, arms, and legs. Her legs also had bilateral pitting oedema and erythema up to her knees. She had a full range of movement of her arms and legs without any

DOI: 10.1201/9781003582007-4

pain. Chest and abdominal examinations were unremarkable. She had a systolic heart murmur.

Her blood pressure was variable, ranging between 93/47 mmHg and 179/65 mmHg during her admission. Due to limited mobility, she was unable to complete a lying and standing blood pressure measurement.

Pulse 72 bpm, temperature 35.1°C, oxygen saturation 96% on air, respiratory rate 16/min, weight 48 kg.

4AT 8/12

Six-Item Screener 0/6

Investigations

Biochemistry	Value	Reference range	Haematology	Value	Reference range
Sodium	134	133–146 mmol/L	Haemoglobin	97	115–165 g/L
Potassium	3.7	3.5–5.3 mmol/L	MCV	102	82–100 fL
Urea	4.3	2.5–7.8 mmol/L	White cell count	2.7	4–11 10^9/L
Creatinine	54	49–90 umol/L	Neutrophils	1.9	2–7.5 10^9/L
C-reactive protein	69	< 5 mg/L	Lymphocytes	0.4	1.5–4 10^9/L
B-type natriuretic peptide	4,931	< 400 ng/L	Platelets	145	140–400 10^9/L
Albumin	34	35–50 g/L	Vitamin B12	949	150–1000 ng/L
TSH	3.4	0.3–4.5 mIU/L	Folate	11.9	2–18.8 ug/L
Vitamin D	89	> 50 nmol/L	Ferritin	45	12–250 ug/L

Viral swab for influenza/COVID was negative.
ECG—sinus rhythm, left bundle branch block
Telemetry performed for first 24 hours of admission, no arrhythmia detected

Echocardiogram: mild-moderate left ventricular hypertrophy and mildly impaired systolic function (ejection fraction 44%). Normal size right ventricle. Normal size atria with mild aortic regurgitation and no aortic stenosis.

Progress

Initial physiotherapy assessment—mobile with two-wheeled walking frame and the assistance of two people.

What could you do about Joan falling over and bruising?

Does she have heart failure?

What would you do about her blood pressure?

How would you change the cardiovascular system medications she takes?

Would you stop or start any other medications?

Is the extensive bruising a sign of elder abuse?

What are the considerations for discharge planning?

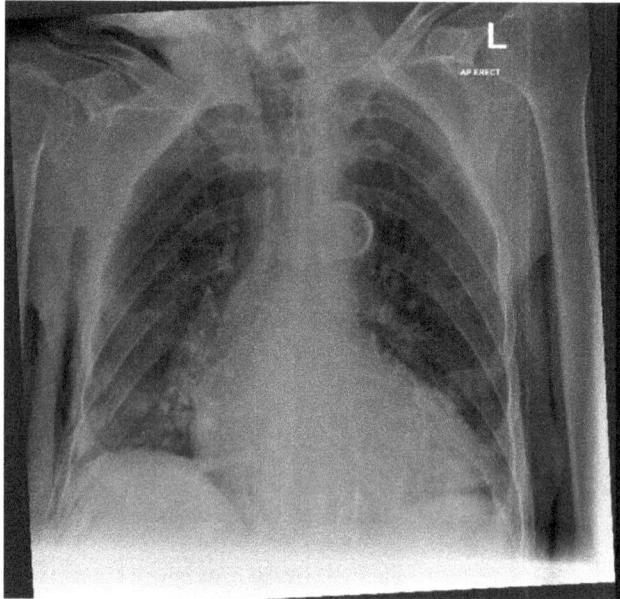

Figure 4.1 Chest X-ray.

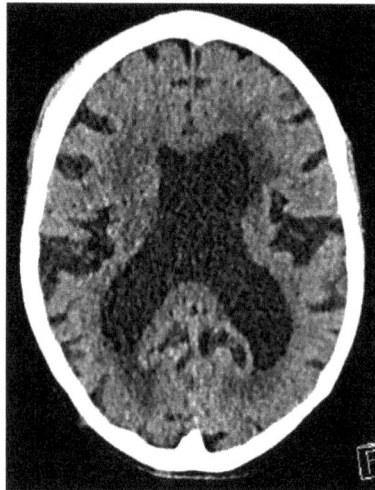

Figure 4.2 CT brain scan showing prominent sulci, enlarged ventricles, and small vessel ischaemic changes (see Figure 2.2).

Falls

There are many possible contributing risk factors for falls, both intrinsic and extrinsic to the person (see Figure 4.3). These can be subdivided into four categories, which are outlined later. Frail older people often have several potential contributors for falling in combination. Identifying these can lead to a holistic management plan. Ambiguous terms, such as

Personal
Cognitive impairment
Reduced vision
Impaired balance

Orthostatic hypotension

Sarcopenia
Arthritis

Peripheral neuropathy
Overgrown toenails

Unsuitable shoes

Environmental
Poorly lit staircase
Single bannister rail

Lack of downstairs toilet

Inappropriate mobility aid

Steps to access property
No hand rails

Loose rugs
Trailing wires

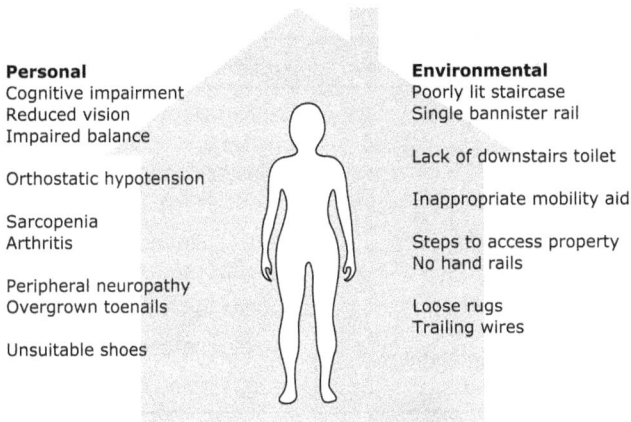

Figure 4.3 Examples of intrinsic and extrinsic risk factors for falls.

'mechanical fall', 'accidental fall', or 'unexplained fall', have no diagnostic value and should be avoided. Falls and syncope (transient loss of consciousness due to globally reduced cerebral blood flow) can be difficult to distinguish in the absence of a witness account. Older people can have amnesia for lost consciousness, and the same pathological mechanisms can contribute to either presentation. Beware of under-evaluating people who say, 'I just tripped'. Try to clarify vague terms like 'dizziness'—did the patient have vertigo, light-headedness, or imbalance? 'Collapse query cause' doesn't narrow things down and is equivalent to saying that the patient is unwell.

Chronic Impairments

Multiple possibilities, examples include visual impairment, peripheral neuropathy, arthritis, and cognitive impairment.

Acute Illnesses

Any acute illness increases the risk of a person with frailty falling over.

Medication Adverse Effects

Drugs that affect the cardiovascular system often increase the risk of orthostatic hypotension (OH). Drugs that affect the neurological system may suppress some brain mechanisms, including balance. This can also be the result of hypoglycaemia. See Table 4.1. In some situations, drugs could reduce the risk of falling, for example, painkillers because an antalgic gait is likely to be unstable.

Environment

Trip hazards around the home can include loose rugs, trailing wires, and poorly lit staircases. The unfamiliarity of novel environments, such as hospital wards, can be hazardous, especially if vision is impaired.

Table 4.1 Medications that Increase the Risk of Falling

Cardiovascular system	Neurological system
Antihypertensives Antianginals Diuretics • Loop diuretics • Mineralocorticoid receptor antagonists • Sodium-glucose co-transporter 2 inhibitors • Angiotensin receptor antagonists with neprilysin inhibitors	Benzodiazepines Opiates Antipsychotics Anticholinergics • e.g. antidepressants, bladder anticholinergics [see Case 9] Dopaminergic medications • e.g. co-careldopa, ropinirole Hypoglycaemics

For Joan, the falls are likely due to a combination of gait and balance problems related to the old stroke and leg oedema, cognitive impairment, there may be an undiagnosed acute illness (e.g. recent functional decline, high C-reactive protein), probably an element of orthostatic hypotension (e.g. variable blood pressure, antihypertensive medication), and there may be environmental hazards in her home that could be detected by an occupational therapist home visit. However, no adjustments to her home will altogether remove the risk of falling. The unfamiliar environment of a hospital ward or care home placement could pose a greater risk to her than returning home. Cognitive impairment increases the risk of falling through a variety of mechanisms. For example, the person may forget about their physical impairment and attempt to move too quickly or without the appropriate mobility aid.

Joan also has an abnormal ECG. It is possible that her falls could be related to a cardiac arrhythmia. Maybe her daughter has witnessed a fall to help us? Cardiac syncope is suggested by the onset of symptoms occurring at rest or during exertion, rather than on standing. An association with chest pain, palpitations, or breathlessness would also make it more likely. Hospital attendance with facial bruising following a fall also increases the chance of syncope being the cause (although people with frailty can lose the self-preservation response of an outstretched hand whilst falling). If there are suggestive features, then a prolonged ECG recording could help.

The assessment of people who have fallen should try to identify potential causes to enable creation of a management plan. Ask about events before and after the fall. What were they doing went it happened? Were there any warning symptoms? Do they remember falling/ hitting the ground? How did they feel afterwards? Could they get themselves up off the floor? When available, a witness account can add helpful details. Cognition should be assessed. Injuries should be identified. All people who have fallen and then can't walk should also have a neurological examination.

OH can contribute to falls and syncope. This can be detected by doing both lying and standing blood pressure measurements. A drop in blood pressure (20 mmHg systolic/10 mmHg diastolic) and/or a feeling of light-headedness on standing is suggestive of OH, but it may not occur every time the person rises. An ECG should be checked. In hospital, patients at risk of falls might be moved to more visible locations on the ward and with increased level of observation. Future fracture risk and bone health should also be considered. Falls nurse specialists can see people with recurrent falls in hospital and access appropriate follow-up.

Bruising

Joan's blood tests show mild macrocytic anaemia, leukopenia, and thrombocytopenia. Although there are several potential causes of this, in her case, myelodysplasia is the most likely. Of note, her vitamin B_{12} and folate were not reduced. Myelodysplasia is an age-related reduction in bone marrow function. It does not usually require any specific treatment.

She is taking clopidogrel for secondary prevention of stroke. The primary event was now 12 years ago. The risk of recurrent stroke is highest in the first year following a stroke and gradually declines over time. In clinical trials for secondary vascular prevention, around 100 people need to be treated with an antiplatelet agent per year to prevent one serious vascular event.[1] Her multiple falls, low platelet count, and bruising all suggest a higher risk from clopidogrel. The long time since her stroke and her reduced life expectancy suggest she may benefit less from continuation. We can discuss this with Joan and her daughter.

Leg Oedema

There are several possible causes of leg oedema (see Table 4.2). Many presentations are multifactorial in older people with frailty. The oedema can be associated with overlying

Table 4.2 Common Causes of Bilateral Leg Swelling in Older People

Cause	Comment
Heart failure	Look for other signs of fluid overload—such as raised JVP or chest X-ray changes Treated with diuretics
Low albumin	Can be caused by renal loss or chronic inflammatory or hepatic disease
Dependent leg oedema (also called gravitational oedema)	Due to gravity plus risk factors Low mobility (especially sleeping in a chair—legs never elevated) Venous insufficiency (associated with hypertension) Treated by elevating legs when possible and/or compression hosiery (N.B. peripheral vascular disease)
Medications • Calcium channel blockers • Dopamine agonists • Pioglitazone • Gabapentin/ pregabalin • NSAIDs • Ranolazine	Discontinuation or switching to an alternative type of medication should be considered
Lymphoedema (non-pitting oedema)	Reduced lymphatic transport Can be associated with obesity May be helped by weight loss or compression bandages

bilateral erythema (N.B. this is not cellulitis, which is a unilateral condition). 'Chronic venous insufficiency' describes a state of sustained venous hypertension caused by valve incompetency and reduced calf muscle pump action, which can lead to 'dependent' (or 'gravitational') oedema. It can be associated with varicose veins, a history of deep vein thrombosis, venous leg ulcers, or obesity. It can precipitate venous eczema, which causes red, dry, itchy, scaling skin. This can be treated with topical emollients but occasionally requires short-term topical steroid use. Lipodermatosclerosis is chronic inflammation and subcutaneous fibrosis caused by venous stasis. The skin can develop brown discolouration due to haemosiderin deposition, and there may be venous ulcers, usually over the ankle malleoli.

In Joan's case, the oedema is likely due to a combination of an adverse effect of lercanidipine, a dependent component due to sleeping in a chair and reduced mobility, and her mildly low serum albumin. Appropriate initial management is to stop lercanidipine, enable her to sleep in a bed, and elevate her legs when possible while sitting.

Heart Failure

Joan has an abnormal ECG and a systolic heart murmur. She also had a raised serum B-type natriuretic peptide (BNP), but the rationale for doing this test is unclear from her presentation. These findings led to her having an echocardiogram. It could be argued that any significant finding on this test may not affect her management, i.e. she would be unlikely to undergo a cardiac valvular procedure, and medications for heart failure that lower blood pressure might be avoided.

Her leg oedema has a more likely alternative explanation than heart failure. There are no other clinical signs, and she doesn't have the typical symptoms of heart failure, such as breathlessness. Sleeping in a chair is likely due to impaired mobility rather than avoiding orthopnoea. This could be clarified with Joan and her daughter. Her ECG is abnormal, and her BNP is raised. BNP is not specific for heart failure and can be elevated by several pathologies and old age. The echocardiogram does show some impairment of systolic function, but her ejection fraction is only mildly reduced at 44%. In geriatric medicine, things are rarely simple. Treating her leg oedema as suggested is a reasonable first approach. A trial of diuretics could be considered if this failed to improve the oedema, especially if carrying the extra fluid around was felt to be contributing to her reduced mobility. However, diuretics could precipitate OH. Similarly, any medication for prognostic benefit in heart failure, such as a sodium-glucose co-transporter 2 inhibitor, could increase her risk of falling.

Blood Pressure

Her blood pressure (BP) has been variable during her admission. High BP can be precipitated by distress or pain. Cognitive impairment may exacerbate this. Regarding her falls and risk of injury, episodes of low BP are of most concern. Frailty is associated with greater risk of medication adverse effects and, due to reduced life expectancy, a lower chance of prognostic benefit. Consequently, guidelines from the National Institute for Health and Care Excellence do not suggest a target BP for people with frailty or multi-morbidity but instead suggest 'use judgement'.[2] Avoiding episodes of low BP is most likely to help reduce her risk of falling.

Starting BP-lowering medications during a hospital admission of non-cardiovascular causation is associated with a greater risk of harm.[3] Performing an out-patient 24-hour BP recording after she has gone home would be an option. However, given her cognitive impairment and reduced mobility, completing the test would have some degree of burden, and the result may not alter management.

Medicines Optimisation

She has been taking alendronate for six years since her hip fracture. Clinical trials have shown that after three to five years of bisphosphonate use, the fracture risk reduction is maintained for the next five years, even if the medication is discontinued.[4] A weekly oral bisphosphonate must be taken in a specific way (in the morning, 30 minutes before any food or other medications, while sitting upright and followed by 200 mls of water). This can be challenging for older people with frailty. Joan's life expectancy is less than five years. Deprescribing the alendronate should be considered. Calcium and vitamin D supplements are unlikely to have much effect alone and could also be considered for stopping.

Like clopidogrel, the benefit of the statin 12 years after her stroke may now be diminished. Possible adverse effects of statins include muscle inflammation and myalgia [see Case 19]. Given her low muscle mass, reduced mobility, and susceptibility to adverse reactions, discontinuation of the statin is also an option to discuss.

She has been on a very low dose of phenytoin for a historical diagnosis of seizures. As the diagnosis was made so long ago, we may not be able to find any details to clarify why a seizure disorder was thought more likely than alternative conditions, such as vasovagal syncope. She hasn't had an event for several decades. For both reasons, the risk of recurrent seizures is low should she discontinue phenytoin. The decision relies on weighing up the possibility of adverse effects from phenytoin, such as falls, against the risk of harms from recurrence of epilepsy. Given Joan's cognitive impairment, her daughter might be able to help with the decision-making process. Checking the serum phenytoin level could aid discussions. If she is well below the therapeutic range on her current dose, then discontinuation would be unlikely to provoke seizures.

Elder Abuse

In Joan's case, her daughter is doing an incredibly good job of providing care for her. There is no suggestion that Joan is being deliberately mistreated. Caring for someone is an important role done 24-hours a day, 365 days a year, often with little acknowledgment. Carers can worry about whether they are doing a good job and deserve words of praise. But this isn't always the case.

Older people can experience neglect, physical, financial, psychological, or sexual mistreatment. Such abuse can be deliberate or accidental (e.g. due to lack of knowledge or support) and may be a sign of carer stress. Transitioning from relative to carer is a challenging task for many people. Harm can occur from acts of omission, such as not seeking appropriate help after a fall. Social isolation and cognitive impairment increase vulnerability. Abusers are most commonly family members, and most abuse occurs in a person's own home. Potential warning signs include delays in seeking medical attention, multiple admissions, inconsistent stories, emotional withdrawal, medication overuse or underuse, multiple injuries of varying age, malnutrition, pressure ulcers, occult fractures, or poor hygiene. Lesions that could indicate physical abuse, rather than accidents, include head and neck injuries (especially the left cheek) in the absence of ones on the limbs. Observing the relationship between patient and carer is helpful. Enquire how the patient feels regarding safety at home. Find out if their carer is properly trained and supported in that role and if they are experiencing stress.

Safeguarding of vulnerable adults is the responsibility of all healthcare professionals. If there is concern raised about potential abuse, it is important to follow local guidelines to share information appropriately with social services colleagues. Interdisciplinary teams are responsible for assessing risk when issues arise and can offer support and training for carers and professionals alike.

What about Joan?

Physiotherapy input helped ensure Joan has the correct walking aid and improved her mobility through techniques and exercises. Other team members incorporated their advice when assisting her on the ward, such as going to the toilet. During the admission, Joan improved to mobilising with a two-wheeled walker and the assistance of one person but didn't manage to do it independently. Further rehabilitation in her own home or attending gait and balance training classes may be suitable for her. An occupational therapist can ensure that she has the appropriate equipment and support at home. In this case, enabling her to sleep in a bed is a key consideration. Options include fitting a bed lever to the side of her current bed or providing a hospital bed for her home. Stairs within a property can be difficult. Possible solutions include fitting a second banister rail, installing a stairlift, or downstairs living. A commode can allow easier toilet access. An occupational therapist home visit can identify and mitigate environmental hazards.

A care package could be provided to assist with personal care. This could also reduce any stress experienced by her daughter. However, some people do not want strangers in their own home, and the timing of visits may not be ideal. For example, a last call in the evening to get someone ready for bed may be several hours before they want to go to bed. Some people with cognitive impairment will lack mental capacity to make informed decisions about their place of residence or care requirements. When this occurs, we need to work as a team, including relatives and carers, to make choices in the patient's best interests. The least restrictive option should be favoured. Always ask your patient what they want, and whenever possible, make this happen.

We should also discuss treatment escalation planning for Joan with her and her daughter. What matters to Joan? Does she prioritise longevity, symptom control, or time at home with her daughter and cats? What are her goals? Would she want to be admitted to hospital again if she had life-threatening illness, or would she and her daughter prefer to aim for palliative care at home?

Key Points

- Falls are often caused by a combination of acute illnesses, chronic conditions that affect gait and balance, medication adverse effects, and environmental hazards.

- Leg oedema has several possible causes—check serum albumin, medications, and mobility.
- During a hospital admission, episodes of low blood pressure are more likely to cause harm than the odd high measurement.
- Carer stress is common and can contribute to the risk of elder abuse.
- Discharge planning usually starts with asking your patient what they want and, whenever possible, making this happen.

Further Reading

1. Antithrombotic Trialists' Collaboration. Aspirin in the primary and secondary prevention of vascular disease: collaborative meta-analysis of individual participant data from randomised trials. *Lancet* 2009;373:1849–60. https://doi.org/10.1016/S0140-6736(09)60503-1

2. *Hypertension in Adults: Diagnosis and Management.* NICE Guideline [NG136]. 2019. www.nice.org.uk/guidance/ng136

3. Anderson TS, Jing B, Auerbach A, et al. Clinical outcomes after intensifying antihypertensive medication regimens among older adults at hospital discharge. *JAMA Intern Med* 2019;179:1528–36. https://doi.org/10.1001/jamainternmed.2019.3007

4. Black DM, Schwartz AV, Ensrud KE, et al. Effects of continuing or stopping alendronate after 5 years of treatment: the Fracture Intervention Trial Long-term Extension (FLEX): A randomized trial. *JAMA* 2006;296:2927–38. https://doi.org/10.1001/jama.296.24.2927

Case 5

Dorothy

Dorothy is an 89-year-old woman who presented to hospital with reduced mobility. On the day of admission, Dorothy's daughter visited and found her mother stuck in a chair. Exactly how long she had been there was unclear but at least a few hours. Her daughter lives over 50 miles away and is the main carer for her disabled son but visits when she can. Dorothy's daughter saw multiple medication packets in several areas around Dorothy's house. There had been a decline in Dorothy's mobility and cognitive function over the past six months. Dorothy hasn't left her home in the last three months.

Past Medical History

Depression
Cognitive impairment (no formal diagnosis of dementia)
Ischaemic heart disease
Type 2 diabetes
COPD
Osteoporosis—wrist fracture eight years ago
Osteoarthritis

Medication

Alendronate 70 mg weekly	Amitriptyline 10 mg at night (for neck pain)
Aspirin 75 mg od	Atorvastatin 40 mg od
Bisoprolol 5 mg od	Calcium/vitamin D one tablet bd
Carbocisteine 750 mg tds	Gliclazide 80 mg bd
Glycerol trinitrate spray as required	Isosorbide mononitrate 20 mg bd
Ivabradine 2.5 mg bd	Lactulose 15 mls bd
Metformin 1 g bd	Mirtazapine 45 mg n
Paracetamol 1 g qds	Salbutamol inhaler as required
Sitagliptin 100 mg od	Umeclidinium with vilanterol (55 mcg/22 mcg) dry powder inhaler (DPI) od

Social History

Dorothy lives alone in a ground floor flat. She mobilises around her flat with a two-wheeled walking frame. She does not have a formal provision of care. Her daughter organises for meals

DOI: 10.1201/9781003582007-5

to be delivered, and neighbours help with any other shopping that she requires. She does not smoke or drink any alcohol these days.

Examination

Heart sounds revealed a soft systolic murmur. There was no peripheral oedema. In the chest, there was mild generalised reduced air entry and expiratory wheeze. Her abdomen was soft and non-tender. No focal neurological deficit was detected.

Six-Item Screener 2/6

4AT 3/12

BP 136/71 mmHg, pulse 64 bpm, oxygen saturation 93% on air, temperature 36.2°C, glucose 9.0 mmol/L

Investigations

Biochemistry	Value	Reference range	Haematology	Value	Reference range
Sodium	141	133–146 mmol/L	Haemoglobin	123	115–165 g/L
Potassium	3.6	3.5–5.3 mmol/L	MCV	87	82–100 fL
Urea	11.3	2.5–7.8 mmol/L	White cell count	5.9	4–11 10^9/L
Creatinine	94	49–90 umol/L	Platelets	354	140–400 10^9/L
C-reactive protein	11	< 5 mg/L			

Liver blood tests and calcium normal

HB_{A1C} 63 mmol/mol a month ago

Chest X-ray—no focal lesion

ECG sinus rhythm, 59 bpm, no ischaemic changes

Would you describe Dorothy's polypharmacy as appropriate?
How could her medication adherence be improved?

Medications

Because long-term conditions accumulate as we age, many older people accumulate medications to control these conditions over their lifespan. Polypharmacy is a term for taking many medications, often considered present for people taking five or more each day. Using this definition, more than half of people aged over 85 in England have polypharmacy.[1]

Rather than focusing on number of medications taken, polypharmacy may be better described as appropriate or inappropriate (problematic). Appropriate polypharmacy is the optimal management of multi-morbidity. In this situation, it is very likely that the benefits of each medication exceed the risk of harm and prescribing is consistent with patient wishes and goals. However, the following are examples of when polypharmacy is likely to be inappropriate:[2]

- The available evidence base doesn't support efficacy for the treatment
- The risk of harm is likely to outweigh the chance of benefit

35

- Hazardous drug combinations
- Unacceptable therapeutic burden to the patient
- Evidence of reduced medication adherence
- Prescribing cascades (i.e. adverse effects caused by a medication are misinterpreted as a new diagnosis leading to the prescription of an additional medication, e.g. furosemide to treat peripheral oedema caused by diltiazem)

Medicines maybe become inappropriate as a clinical picture evolves. For example, statins for vascular prevention for someone who is close to the end of life due to advanced dementia, or renally excreted medicines for someone who has developed severe renal impairment. Sometimes a non-pharmacological approach would be better than prescribing, for example, mobilising someone to the toilet rather than requiring laxatives to use a bedpan. Medication review is a key component of geriatric care and should aim to eradicate inappropriate polypharmacy.

Adverse Drug Reactions

It has been calculated that adverse drug reactions (ADR) are the cause of or a contributing factor to around one in six hospital admissions.[3] This figure could be higher for older people with frailty, especially if the ADR presents in a less obvious way, e.g. contributing to falls or cognitive impairment. Always consider medication effects in your differential diagnosis. ADR more commonly affect people with polypharmacy and can be due to interactions between medications, with medications and other morbidities, or due to the physiological effects of biological ageing (i.e. frailty is state of increased vulnerability):

- Drug-drug interactions—e.g. increased bleeding with aspirin and apixaban co-prescribed
- Drug-disease interactions—e.g. increased peripheral oedema with amlodipine and heart failure
- Drug-frailty interactions—e.g. increased risk of cognitive impairment with anticholinergic medications due to increased permeability of the blood-brain barrier

Some drugs have high incidences of ADR in frail older people and are only rarely appropriate, e.g. benzodiazepines, anticholinergics, non-steroidal anti-inflammatory drugs (NSAIDs), and antipsychotics.

Adherence

Reliably following a complex schedule of medicines is difficult. The World Health Organisation has estimated that only half of medicines are consistently taken as prescribed.[4] Taking medications as prescribed requires both motivation and capability. Low motivation leads to intentional non-adherence. Examples include prescribing not being aligned with patient goals or the patient experiencing/worry about developing an ADR. Capability to take a medicine requires remembering, accessible packaging, and an appropriate drug formulation. For example, liquid medications may be better for some people with swallowing difficulties, and available types of inhaler suit people differently [see Case 22]. Switching to a longer acting formulation of a medication that needs to be taken less frequently could also help. Medication adherence may be reduced at home but then given as prescribed during a hospital admission or change of care environment. Alternatively, medications usually taken may be omitted due to inaccurate information about current prescription or medication unavailability. Either scenario can result in patient harm.

Optimising medication adherence requires attention to motivation and capability. Ensure prescribing aligns with their goals, detect ADR or concern about their development, and educate about potential benefits of adherence. Capability is improved by simplifying regimes, i.e. fewer medicines and/or fewer doses. Inappropriate polypharmacy should be identified and addressed. Reminders can help with memory impairment, such as smartphone alarms. Ensure packaging is accessible. Carers can assist with medication-taking. Ensure the best formulation is provided. Check inhaler technique. Multi-dose administration aids can help in some situations but have limitations. Some medications can't be placed in them, for example, insulin, liquids, inhalers, and medications taken in a specific way (e.g. bisphosphonates). Taking medications out of their packets removes the associated information leaflets. Individual tablets become hard to identify. This can affect 'sick day rules', such as the ability to omit a laxative when suffering from diarrhoea.

What about Dorothy?

Initial assessments have not found a clear cause for Dorothy's presentation. There has been a progressive decline in physical and cognitive function over recent months. She is developing frailty (CFS 5) and is at risk of harm, such as a fall with injury or long lie on the floor. There is a suggestion that medication adherence has declined. She is prescribed 16 different regular medications.

We need to obtain some more information to assess whether this polypharmacy is appropriate, mainly by speaking to Dorothy and possibly with her daughter's help. We need to ensure we have an accurate list of her current medicines, know why each one was prescribed, and how long she has been taking them. What are her personal goals and wishes? Does she get symptomatic benefit from the medicines? Has she experienced/is she worried about ADR? Does she feel a sense of therapeutic burden? Does she have the physical and cognitive ability to take the medicines? Regarding medications taken for long-term disease prevention, we need to consider her life expectancy. We also need to set appropriate therapeutic targets (e.g. blood pressure and glucose control). We need to look for drug-drug, drug-disease, and drug-frailty interactions, as well as prescribing cascades. Is she prescribed the optimal dose and formulation for each drug?

Given Dorothy's complex history and lengthy prescription list, medicines optimisation will take skill and time. It may need to be done gradually over several occasions and with good communication and review to look for re-emergence of symptoms or drug withdrawal effects. We might start by thinking about amitriptyline because it has anticholinergic effects that could worsen her cognition. She is also prescribed another antidepressant, i.e. mirtazapine. If there is no clear ongoing symptomatic benefit for neck pain, then a trial without is justified. Given her mobility has declined, she may no longer get angina. Perhaps a withdrawal of isosorbide or ivabradine could be tried? Does she get symptomatic benefit from carbocisteine, maybe also try without [see Case 22]? Alendronate is difficult to take, and because she has taken it for several years, she may not get any future benefit [see Case 4]. What is her target for glucose control? She may not need three antidiabetic medications to achieve this and is at risk from hypoglycaemia [see Case 10]. We should continue working through the list to consider each of her medications in turn. Fewer tablets will reduce the risk of ADR, non-adherence, and therapeutic burden.

It is worth considering whether we think she has been taking her medicines at all. If not, then restarting them all at the time of admission would be quite risky. In this situation, it is often wise to avoid prescribing all usual medications but instead look to reduce swiftly. This can be done by reducing each group of medicines to a safe minimum (e.g. not three anti-diabetic medications but instead give one [or none] and monitor the blood sugars over the first day or two). A good option is suspending all the long-term risk reduction medicines that do not have withdrawal syndromes in the initial prescription while pharmacy colleagues explore with community counterparts to work out if prescriptions have been filled and a clearer picture emerges. Building the appropriate prescription back up does not need to be rushed.

Dorothy needs CGA delivered by a multi-disciplinary team. Physiotherapy can help optimise her mobility and use of the correct walking aid. Occupational therapy can assess her function and provide useful home adaptations. Pharmacists can help with medicine optimisation. Social services can help to arrange any required package of care. A referral to the local memory clinic could help establish a diagnosis for her cognitive impairment and ensure she has the right management and support.

Key Points

- Medication review is a key component of geriatric care and should aim to eradicate inappropriate polypharmacy.
- Always consider if a patient's symptom/presentation could be caused, or contributed to, by an adverse drug effect.
- Reduced medication adherence is very common and may fluctuate with a change in care environment.
- Ask patients how they feel about their medications. Do they feel that the benefit exceeds the burden for each drug?
- Communicate any prescription changes made to the patient and their primary care team.

Further Reading

1. *Health Survey for England 2016: Prescribed Medicines.* files.digital.nhs.uk/pdf/3/c/hse2016-pres-med.pdf

2. Duerden M, Avery T, Payne R. *Polypharmacy and Medicines Optimisation: Making it Safe and Sound.* 2013. The King's Fund. www.kingsfund.org.uk

3. Osanlou R, Walker L, Hughes DA, et al. Adverse drug reactions, multimorbidity and polypharmacy: a prospective analysis of 1 month of medical admissions. *BMJ Open* 2022;12:e055551. https://doi.org/10.1136/bmjopen-2021–055551

4. World Health Organization. *Adherence to Long-Term Therapies: Evidence for Action.* 2003. World Health Organization. https://apps.who.int/iris/handle/10665/42682

Case 6

Sarah

Sarah is an 83-year-old retired shop worker who came to hospital after a fall at home. She couldn't recall this event. Her son thought she must have gone outside to her garden to bring in laundry from the washing line. Then, presumably, she tripped and fell over. She is usually mobile independently around her property but rarely goes out. Her son noticed a golf-ball-sized lump on her head and phoned for an ambulance. After initial assessment, she was brought to the emergency department. There had been no witnessed loss of consciousness, vomiting, or seizures.

Three weeks before, blood tests done by her GP had found hyponatraemia (sodium 120). Her GP visited her at home, in the company of her daughter, and explained why going to hospital could be helpful. She said that she felt fine and was adamant that she would not go to hospital for any investigations regardless of risk. Three years previously, she had complained of chest pain and had a CT pulmonary angiogram to exclude a pulmonary embolus. This scan had found an incidental 10 mm nodule in her right lung apex. She has smoked 20 to 40 cigarettes per day for many decades. She was seen in the respiratory medicine clinic but declined any further follow-up or chest imaging, even though she was aware it could be an early lung cancer. She also did not want to consider stopping smoking. Her son reported that she stopped taking all her tablets about two months ago.

Past Medical History

COPD
Type 2 diabetes
Anxiety/depression

Medication

Beclometasone with formoterol and glycopyrronium inhaler 87/5/9 two puffs bd	Salbutamol inhaler PRN

She was prescribed other medications until recently but hadn't been taking any of them for the last two months: aspirin 75 mg od, atorvastatin 20 mg od, bumetanide 1 mg od, citalopram 10 mg od, metformin 1 g bd, and perindopril 6 mg od.

DOI: 10.1201/9781003582007-6

Social History

Sarah lives alone and rarely leaves the house. Her family and neighbours support with shopping and laundry, but she is otherwise independent. She doesn't use any walking aids. There is a banister rail on each side of her staircase.

Physical Examination

Chest examination revealed mild wheeze throughout but no crackles and equal air entry. Heart sounds were normal, and there was no peripheral oedema. Jugular venous pressure (JVP) was normal. Her abdomen was soft and non-tender. Clinical examination did not suggest she had a skull fracture.

Six-Item Screener 3/6

4AT 3/12

BP 127/76 mmHg, pulse 72 bpm, oxygen saturation 95% on air, temperature 36.2°C, glucose 8.4 mmol/L

Investigations

Biochemistry	Value	Reference range	Haematology	Value	Reference range
Sodium	121	133–146 mmol/L	Haemoglobin	119	115–165 g/L
Potassium	4.6	3.5–5.3 mmol/L	MCV	82	82–100 fL
Urea	4.2	2.5–7.8 mmol/L	White cell count	6.2	4–11 10^9/L
Creatinine	62	49–90 umol/L	Platelets	257	140–400 10^9/L
C-reactive protein	13	< 5 mg/L			
TSH	1.7	0.3–4.5 mIU/L			
Serum osmolality	256	275–295 mosmol/kg			

Sodium 120 three weeks ago but in the normal range three months ago
Urine sodium 12 mmol/L, urine potassium 53 mmol/L, urine osmolality 306 mosmol/kg
HbA1c 46 mmol/mol three weeks ago
CT scan of brain—no focal abnormality detected

Progress

When the initial test results were available, the emergency department doctor returned to plan the next steps. Sarah was agitated and said she wanted to go home. The doctor asked her to recap her admission so far. She said she is confused and was brought in for this reason. She said she fell over and thought it was while doing the ironing. She recalled her GP visiting her at home in recent weeks. The doctor explained that her GP had been worried about her low sodium, and tests that day showed the same problem, which could provoke seizures and be life-threatening. In response, she said she would eat more salt. The doctor explained that it

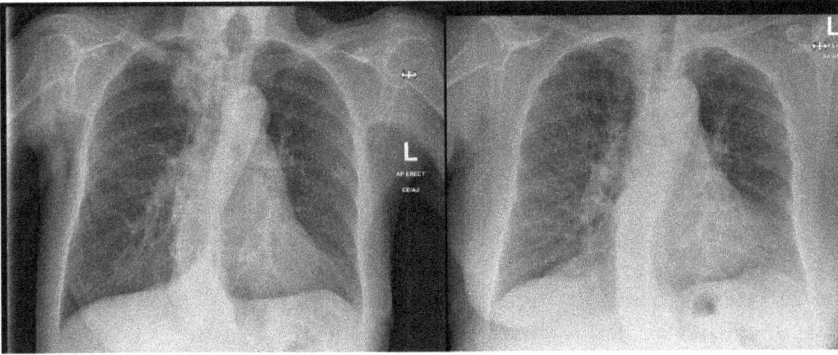

Figure 6.1 Chest X-ray at the time of admission showing a mass near the right lung apex and from three years ago for comparison.

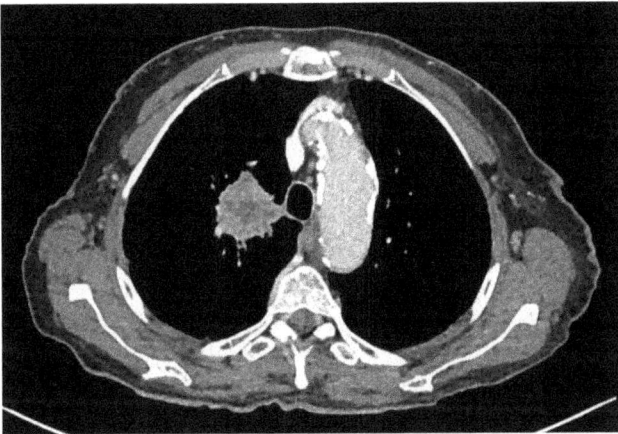

Figure 6.2 CT scan of chest showing a mass in the upper zone of the right lung.

is not that simple, and there could be various causes, including some tumours. The patient said she wanted to go home, sit on her sofa, and watch television. When asked to recap the conversation, she shouted, 'I don't know what you said because I don't remember!' Given her lack of recall, it was judged that she did not have capacity to decide to leave hospital.

The doctor then spoke to the patient's son. Her son was concerned that his mother would be very agitated if she had to stay in hospital, partly because she wants to smoke regularly. The doctor said she was very low in sodium and required treatment. Her son still wondered if she should go home because she always got distressed in hospital, and she has previously shared wishes to be cared for at home if approaching the end of life. The doctor explained that she lacked capacity to decide for herself and so was going to be admitted to a medical ward.

What is the likely cause of her hyponatraemia?
What is the treatment of her hyponatraemia?
How do we establish if she has mental capacity to make decisions?
How do we know what is in her best interests?

Hyponatraemia

The evaluation of hyponatraemia can be over-complicated by assessment algorithms that start with test results and work back towards the patient. As with other conditions, start with taking a history and doing an examination, only then move on to test results. In older people, the cause can be multifactorial.

History should establish recent symptoms, fluid intake, and medications. Examination should evaluate volume status. Syndrome of inappropriate antidiuretic hormone secretion (SIADH) causes excess renal water reabsorption despite decreased plasma osmolality (i.e. urine is inappropriately concentrated). SIADH can be precipitated by medications, respiratory, and intracranial disorders. Common culprit medications are antidepressants and carbamazepine. Common causes of hyponatraemia are compared in Table 6.1. Frequently requested additional tests are discussed later. Hypothyroidism and adrenocortical deficiency are rarer causes of hyponatraemia.

Serum Osmolality

Serum sodium concentration is the main determinant of osmolality. So, serum osmolality is usually low when serum sodium is low. The exception being when a lot of a different substance is present. With severe hyperglycaemia, serum osmolality can be > 295 mosm/kg. Less commonly, raised serum protein (e.g. myeloma) or lipid (e.g. triglyceride) concentrations can cause hyponatraemia with a normal serum osmolality.

Urine Osmolality

Our kidneys control the composition of urine to preserve homeostasis. In usual conditions, they create urine that is more concentrated than our serum (500–850 mosm/kg over 24 hours), but depending on fluid intake, random urine samples can vary in the

Table 6.1 Common Causes of Hyponatraemia Compared

	SIADH	Excess sodium loss	Fluid overload
History	Symptoms suggesting underlying lung or intracerebral disease Medications—e.g. antidepressants, carbamazepine	*Renal loss* Medications— diuretics; renal disease *Non-renal loss* History of diarrhoea/ vomiting, burns	Heart failure Low serum protein—e.g. renal or gastrointestinal loss; liver disease
Examination	Appear normovolaemic	Normovolaemic or underfilled	Hypervolaemia
Other test results	Urea likely to be normal	Urea may be raised	Albumin may be low
Notes	Likely to improve with fluid restriction	May need intravenous saline infusion	Treat underlying condition

range of 50 to 1200 mosm/kg. With serum hyponatraemia, urine osmolality is usually greater than serum osmolality unless there is very high fluid intake, i.e. polydipsia or beer potomania. These can usually be established from the history and observing the patient.

Urine Sodium

With bodily sodium depletion, urine sodium < 20 mmol/L suggests extra-renal losses (e.g. diarrhoea, vomiting, or burns) and urine sodium > 20 mmol/L suggests renal losses (e.g. diuretic use, renal disease). This distinction may already be obvious clinically. In other situations, urine sodium is unlikely to be helpful.

Sarah has no history of vomiting, diarrhoea, or burns to suggest extra-renal losses. She was taking bumetanide (renal salt loss) and citalopram (a cause of SIADH) in the past, but she stopped taking both two months ago. Examination did not show signs of fluid overload (e.g. peripheral oedema, raised JVP) or dehydration (e.g. raised pulse and low BP). Initial blood tests don't suggest dehydration (e.g. urea in normal range). Despite not taking her diabetes medication, her blood glucose is in the normal range, and her Hb_{A1C} is ok. Her serum osmolality is low, and her urine osmolality is, inappropriately, higher. For Sarah, SIADH is the most likely cause of hyponatraemia, and lung cancer is its most likely precipitant. Limiting her fluid intake to less than 1.5 L/day is the initial treatment. From what we know about Sarah, it is unlikely that she would want to pursue a definitive diagnosis or explore treatment options for the lung cancer.

Mental Capacity

In England and Wales, the term 'mental capacity' relates to the ability to reliably make and communicate a decision.[1] Capacity is decision specific. You may be able to choose some things for yourself but not others. For example, a person may be able to make 'small' decisions, such as what to have for lunch, but not 'big' ones, such as where to live. Also, capacity can change over time. It should be assessed at the point that the relevant decision needs to be made. Sometimes decisions can be postponed until the person has the best chance of participating. Appropriate assistance should also be given to maximise their chance to participate. The process balances the right of a person to make their own decisions against the risk of harm if they fail to protect themselves.

There are five statutory principles:

1. Assume the person has the capacity unless there is reason to suspect not. For example, do they have cognitive impairment (e.g. dementia/delirium)?
2. People should not be treated as unable to decide unless all practicable steps to help them have been tried without success, i.e. correct language, non-verbal communication, treat delirium (unless it is an emergency).
3. A person is not to be treated as unable to decide merely because they make an unwise decision.
4. A decision made on behalf of a person who lacks capacity must be in their best interests.
5. Where possible, the least restrictive option should be chosen for someone who lacks capacity.

Typically, assessment would involve providing the relevant information and options. These should be communicated in the most appropriate way and at the best time. Three questions are relevant. Do they understand the information and consequences, i.e. the nature of the decision, the reason why it is required, and the likely effects of each option? Can they retain the information for long enough to weight up the options/outcomes? Can they communicate their decision (by any means)? If not, then the person lacks capacity, and this decision should be made on their behalf.

Best Interests

Establishing what is in a person's best interests is not always obvious, and there can be disagreement between people involved. The person should be enabled to participate in the decision where possible. Their views should be established, including their past expressions, beliefs, and values. People close to them should be consulted (e.g. relatives, close friends, carers) to identify any previously expressed views. Sometimes, when a person close to them can't be identified, an independent mental capacity advocate can help. When possible, the least restrictive option should be selected. The process is not applicable in some scenarios, e.g. an advance decision to refuse the relevant treatment was previously made at a time when they had capacity to do so.

What about Sarah?

When Sarah arrived on the medical ward, several hours after coming to hospital, she was very distressed. She repeatedly asked why she was being detained because she was just visiting. She continually tried to stand up and walk out. She pushed away anyone who tried to stop her. Another conversation was had with her son. The most likely underlying diagnosis was lung cancer. She had previously declined investigations or interventions three years ago when she had no cognitive impairment. It was agreed that going home was likely to be in her best interests with community palliative care input going forwards.

Key Points

- The cause of hyponatraemia is usually identified from history, examination, and medications.
- Mental capacity to make decisions needs to be established for people with cognitive impairment.
- A 'best interests' decision may be made for someone who lacks mental capacity; the least restrictive option should be favoured.

Further Reading

1. Mental Capacity Act (MCA). 2005. www.gov.uk/government/publications/mental-capacity-act-code-of-practice

Case 7

Pamela

An 86-year-old woman, called Pamela, was brought into hospital by her daughter and daughter-in-law after an unwitnessed fall at her home. Pamela couldn't recall the event. She has a diagnosis of mixed dementia. Her daughter said that she had been more confused and unsteady on her feet over the past two weeks. Initially, it was thought that she may have a UTI and was given an antibiotic by her usual doctor (fosfomycin 3 g granules as a single dose), but this hadn't improved things. Her family were also arranging a dentist appointment to check out a tooth that had been bothering her. On the day of admission, her daughter-in-law found her on the floor near the fireplace in the front room when she visited. Pamela had a cut and bruising around the left side of her forehead. Now in hospital, Pamela does not know why she is here and doesn't have any symptoms.

Past Medical History

Mixed dementia (Alzheimer's and vascular)

Falls: two admissions in last year—rib fractures with one and a traumatic sub-arachnoid haemorrhage with the other

Fractured left neck of femur eight years ago

Medication

Alendronate 70 mg weekly on a Saturday	Aspirin 75 mg od
Calcium and vitamin D one tablet bd	Cyanocobalamin 50 mcg od
Diclofenac topical gel as required	Ferrous sulfate 200 mg od
Lansoprazole 15 mg od	Memantine 20 mg od
Paracetamol 500 mg qds	Simvastatin 40 mg n

Social History

Pamela lives alone in a house and has the support of carers three times a day. Her carers help her with getting washed and dressed, meal preparation, and with taking her medication. They also assist her going up and down the stairs when she gets up in the morning and when going to bed at night. Either her daughter or daughter-in-law also visits every day. She has a two-wheeled walking frame both upstairs and downstairs, but she sometimes forgets to use them.

DOI: 10.1201/9781003582007-7

Examination

Pamela obeyed commands intermittently; sometimes she said she didn't want to. There was a small bruise near her left eyebrow and mild swelling and tenderness around her left lower jaw. Chest was clear and heart sounded normal. Her abdomen was soft and non-tender. Unable to fully examine her neurological system due to reduced engagement but she moved all four limbs against gravity without any obvious asymmetry. Pupils were equal and reactive to light. She had no pain on the internal or external rotation of either hip.

Six-Item Screener 1/6

4AT 8/12

BP 142/83 mmHg, pulse 92 bpm, oxygen saturation 95% on air, temperature 37.0°C, glucose 7.2 mmol/L, weight 49.3 kg.

Lying BP 116/68 mmHg and recording one minute after standing 135/73 mmHg

Investigations

Biochemistry	Value	Reference range	Haematology	Value	Reference range
Sodium	131	133–146 mmol/L	Haemoglobin	116	115–165 g/L
Potassium	4.5	3.5–5.3 mmol/L	MCV	93	82–100 fL
Urea	7.3	2.5–7.8 mmol/L	White cell count	16.3	4–11 10^9/L
Creatinine	77	49–90 umol/L	Platelets	302	140–400 10^9/L
C-reactive protein	66	< 5 mg/L	Vitamin B$_{12}$	149	150–1000 ng/L
Albumin	43	35–50 g/L	Folate	14.3	2–18.8 ug/L
Adjusted calcium	2.49	2.2–2.6 mmol/L	Ferritin	18	12–250 ug/L

Liver blood tests normal
Viral swab for influenza/COVID was negative

ECG—sinus rhythm, 94 bpm

Chest X-ray—no focal lesion

CT head—mild to moderate small vessel ischaemic changes and cerebral atrophy

Progress

Pamela was treated with antibiotics for an infection of suspected dental source on the left side. Her delirium settled over the next three days, and her family felt she was back to her normal self. She previously had a 'do not attempt resuscitation' form. It was confirmed with Pamela and her family that this remained appropriate.

What are the potential risks of alendronate treatment, and how long should it continue?

Should Pamela continue aspirin and simvastatin to slow progression of vascular dementia?

What are the considerations for discharge planning?
What is 'discharge to assess', and would it be useful for Pamela?

Bisphosphonates

Possible complications of prolonged bisphosphonate use include atypical femoral fractures and osteonecrosis of the jaw. Both are rare at the doses of bisphosphonates used for osteoporosis treatment (< 1 per 1000 per year of exposure). However, Pamela currently has a problem with her tooth, which increases the risk of osteonecrosis. For safety reasons, at least withholding alendronate until this is addressed is appropriate.

Pamela has been prescribed alendronate since her hip fracture eight years ago. Bisphosphonates bind to bone and have a half-life of many years. Studies that have compared continuation of bisphosphonates to discontinuation after a period of three to five years have found little difference in fracture occurrence over the next three years. Due to her degree of frailty and co-morbidities, Pamela's life expectancy is less than three years. Permanently discontinuing alendronate is unlikely to increase her fracture risk. Also, alendronate must be taken in a specific way [see Case 4], which could be difficult or burdensome for her. If no longer taking alendronate, the rationale for taking a calcium and vitamin D supplement is less clear. Discontinuation of this medication should also be considered.

Vascular Dementia

There is no clinical trial evidence to suggest that either antiplatelet drugs or statins reduce the progression of vascular dementia. Pamela doesn't have any other known reason to be prescribed these medications. Frailty places her at a higher risk of bleeding complications with aspirin and muscle symptoms with simvastatin. She has mild normocytic anaemia with a borderline low ferritin. The combination of aspirin and alendronate increases her risk of peptic ulceration. She is also prescribed oral iron supplementation. If no longer taking aspirin and alendronate, she may no longer need to take iron and may eventually also be able to also stop lansoprazole.

Discharge Planning

Whereas getting to a hospital is thankfully relatively easy, you can call an ambulance or attend an emergency department, leaving hospital can be much more complicated. Older people with frailty often have a functional decline around an acute illness. Recognising the extent of this change and recovery trajectory can be tricky. Medical practitioners can be poor at describing barriers to discharge and sometimes resort to vague terms like 'needs a full social sort-out'. It is important to identify the specific reasons why a person is still in hospital to be able to identify the best solution.

Older people are at risk of other people making subjective decisions about them without their involvement. The following are a couple of examples of the type of language that is sometimes used:

- 'She can't go home because the ambulance crew said her home was cluttered'.
- 'He can't go home because his daughter has concerns'.

In its basic form, discharge planning involves asking the patient what they want to happen and then making that happen. Sometimes going home is labelled 'unsafe'. In this scenario, it is important to establish specifically why going home is unsafe and for whom. Nothing in life is 100% safe. A reasonable concern could be fear that the patient will fall at home and be unable to get up. This must be taken in context with other risks, such as a reduction in independence while in hospital. Table 7.1 shows examples of common risks to be weighed up when considering discharge from hospital. For people who lack capacity to decide on discharge destination, it must be established what is in their best interests, with the least restrictive option being favoured [see Case 6].

Various team members can assist with discharge planning. Three of the key roles are briefly outlined later, but at times, many others will be needed. Figures 7.1 and 7.2 show some common mobility aids and equipment that can be provided for use at home.

- Physiotherapy—mobility, mobility aids, stair practice
- Occupational therapy—equipment for home, transfers, bathing, care needs
- Social work—care packages, care homes, funding/financial decisions

Table 7.1 Balancing the Risks of Remaining in Hospital or Going Home

Hospital	Home
Hospital-acquired infection	Fall and can't get up
Falls with injury	Periods without care
Deconditioning	No rapid medical review
Restricted liberty	Medication-taking not supervised
Delirium	Financial costs to individual
Pressure ulcers	

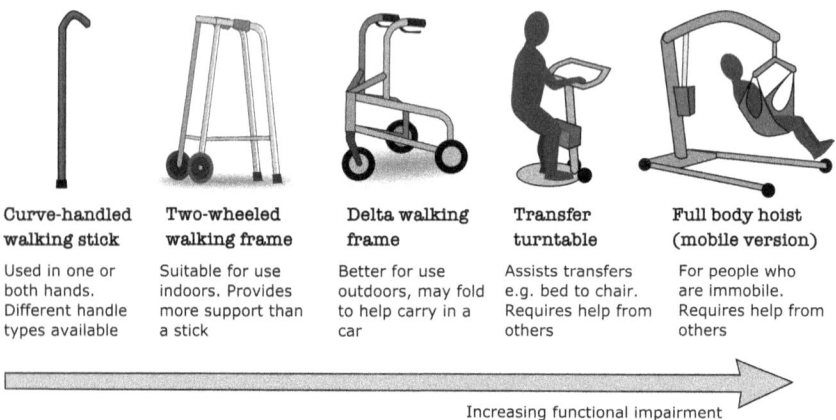

Curve-handled walking stick	Two-wheeled walking frame	Delta walking frame	Transfer turntable	Full body hoist (mobile version)
Used in one or both hands. Different handle types available	Suitable for use indoors. Provides more support than a stick	Better for use outdoors, may fold to help carry in a car	Assists transfers e.g. bed to chair. Requires help from others	For people who are immobile. Requires help from others

Increasing functional impairment

Figure 7.1 Examples of mobility aids.

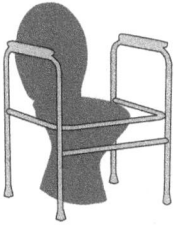

Toilet surround
Makes it easier to get
on and off the toilet

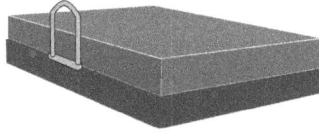

Bed lever
Base slots between mattress
and bed frame. Provides
support getting in/out of bed

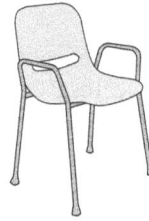

Shower chair
Adjustable height chair
that allows sitting down
while showering

Figure 7.2 Examples of equipment that can help people function more independently at home.

Place of Care

When possible, most people who have been admitted from their own property will want to return to living there. For people with impaired mobility, important considerations are access (e.g. steps up to the front door) and if there are stairs within the property. Having a downstairs toilet limits the number of times a day the stairs must be tackled. A commode could be provided downstairs, or by the bedside to make toileting access easier. Handheld urinals designed for men or women and the use of bedpans are possible alternative solutions. Stairlifts can be installed to improve access. These can sometimes be rented. Getting permission from a landlord could be an issue if the property is not their own. Living downstairs can be an option if space allows. This may require moving a bed into the living room and isn't always acceptable, especially if the property is shared with others. Space in the property can also limit the use of equipment, such as a wheelchair, transfer aid, or full-body hoist. Clutter may also be a tricky issue. A person's life possessions can't simply be thrown out to create space. It must be approached sensitively to gain their agreement.

Sheltered accommodation is usually provided in purpose-built flats that are on the ground floor or have an access lift. A manager or warden is on site some of the time. The accommodation usually has some communal areas, such as a lounge and laundry room. 'Extra sheltered' accommodation usually provides carers for every resident.

Moving into a care home is a big decision. It often has financial implications and can lead to selling a property and parting with most possessions. The new residence becomes their home, and they must feel valued and wanted in it. Choosing the right home is important. In the UK, care homes are subdivided, with some homes providing more than one category. Residential care homes can support all activities of daily living but do not have nurses continually present. Nursing homes have a registered nurse on site and can provide more complex care, such as dressings and administering insulin. Dementia specialist homes (the old term 'elderly mentally infirm' [EMI] is sometimes heard) can care for people with dementia who exhibit challenging behaviours. It is important to consider why a care home is the best option. For example, moving into a care home doesn't stop people falling over, but there may be someone there to help them get up afterwards.

Respite care is sometimes used to help relieve carer stress. It can either be for a few hours a week at a day centre or residential for a period of a week or two. When residential, people with dementia can find it hard to adapt to new environments. Consequently, carer stress may be reduced during the stay but transiently increased afterwards.

49

Carers

Family members often also act as carers. This can be an overwhelming or intimidating additional role. There is a risk that they will experience strain, which has negative implications for the carer and can lead to lower quality care being delivered. In the UK, the usual 'maximum' of care that can be provided by social services is two carers for 30 minutes four times a day. This leaves long periods between visits. Care packages are not always acceptable to individuals. Some people do not like having strangers in their own home. People with cognitive impairment may lack insight into their needs and decline assistance. Sometimes the timing of carer arrival doesn't match with the person's lifestyle, e.g. the last call each day arriving before they want to go to bed.

Final Preparations for Home

Several other steps need to be completed just before going home. Do they have a key to get in, or will someone else be at home? Is the heating on, and is there food in the fridge? Has the care package been restarted? Are their medications ready? Has transport been arranged? Is a referral to the district nurse service required (e.g. dressings, insulin)? Is a follow-up appointment required? Has the discharge letter been completed to ensure good communication with community teams?

Discharge to Assess

'Discharge to assess' (D2A) is a process that allows assessment of function and future needs to occur in a person's own property, using their own equipment. D2A teams can usually provide any extra equipment, arrange home adaptations, and have access to carer support when needed. In case the D2A process demonstrates an unexpected safety risk, then a backup plan of returning to hospital, a rehabilitation unit, or a short-term care placement should be in place. D2A provides a more genuine picture than could be obtained in hospital. It can also speed up discharge, which is beneficial for both sides. There may be other advantages. For example, without seeing someone in their own home, it is difficult to determine where best to place grab rails because the specific location of each patient's hand placement is individual and hard to accurately estimate.

Pamela was assessed by the physiotherapy team and found to be at her baseline mobility, which is independent with a walking frame. Her daughter-in-law described longstanding fluctuations in both her cognition and mobility. At times, she can safely manage stairs; at other times, she cannot. Pamela's family have noticed a marked deterioration in her overall wellbeing over recent months. They expressed concerns around her home environment and the need for adaptations or equipment to maintain independence at home. She was judged appropriate for D2A to assess her in her own environment and identify any outstanding needs. A morning ambulance was arranged given the concerns about fluctuating mobility in case Pamela could not manage the steps to access her property. Pamela's daughter-in-law arranged to be at the property at the time of discharge to allow entry.

By visiting Pamela's property, the D2A team gained much more detail. Her privately-owned house has two steps at the front door to access the porch and an additional step into hallway, with a wall-mounted grab rail. Pamela can manage the steps with assistance and does not go out alone. There is a downstairs toilet, accessed through the kitchen. It is a small space but was big enough to accommodate a free-standing toilet frame, which the D2A team provided. The main bathroom is upstairs; there is a walk-in shower with shower seat and grab rail. There is a straight flight of stairs to a small landing, followed by a 90-degree turn and further three steps to the top landing. There are banister rails on both sides of the stairs. Pamela's daughter-in-law thought she would benefit from an additional grab rail at the top of the stairs because she would normally reach round to get her walking frame, which looks unsafe. This additional rail was requested and would be fitted within 48 hours. Pamela's carers already assisted her on the stairs and could continue to do this until the grab rail was fitted, i.e. no need to return to the hospital ward while awaiting installation. There is a grab rail along the hallway from her bedroom to the bathroom, which she uses when going to the toilet overnight. The provision of commode for the bedside was discussed, but Pamela's daughter said that Pamela had declined this in the past.

Pamela has carers who visit three times a day: morning, teatime, and bedtime. The morning carers make a snack to have for lunch, but Pamela's family have noticed that this is often untouched and think she would also benefit from a lunchtime call. Currently, Pamela is at home alone between 9 AM and 5 PM. The social worker arranged the additional call, increasing her care to four times a day. This package was started at the time of the return home with the D2A team. The carers support all daily activities, including transfers in and out of bed and using the stairs in the morning and bedtime. During the day, Pamela is encouraged to not use the stairs unassisted. Pamela's daughter-in-law thinks she largely obeys this instruction, although there have been occasions when the carers found her already downstairs when they arrived in the morning. She was also provided with a personal care alarm that can be worn like a necklace and activated if she falls and can't get herself up.

What about Pamela?

Pamela has moderate frailty (CFS 6) and remains at high risk of future falls. Her cognitive impairment means that she sometimes forgets to use the walking aid or attempts the stairs without assistance. She has had several prior falls with significant injuries. The home adaptations and increased care can reduce the risk a little, but no reasonable intervention can make things risk free. Her trajectory is one of physical and cognitive decline. It may not be possible to support her at home for much longer, but currently, it is felt to be in her best interests to try. Certainly, this is what she wants. She is lucky to have the excellent support of her family.

Key Points

- When planning a discharge, start by asking people what they want.
- Ask yourself why is this person still in hospital. What are the specific barriers to going home?
- Favour the least restrictive option.
- Avoid a 'safety first' approach. Nothing in life is 100% safe.
- There is no such thing as a 'full social sort out'.

Gordon

Gordon is an 81-year-old retired plumber who had an unwitnessed fall around 8 PM that evening. He was found on the floor in his own room by staff at the care home where he lives. The fall caused a skin tear to his left forearm, which was dressed at the care home prior to coming to hospital. He has also reported right hip pain since the fall. Gordon couldn't recall the details of how he came to fall but thinks he must have tripped. He says he lives with his brother and sister-in-law. He is not in discomfort while lying still. He does not report any other symptoms. The care home staff had not noticed any change in his health over the last few days.

Past Medical History

Iron-deficiency anaemia
Ischaemic heart disease—myocardial infarction 18 months ago, coronary artery bypass
    graft ten years ago
Benign prostatic hyperplasia—long-term urinary catheter
Recurrent UTI
Vascular dementia/cerebrovascular disease
Atrial fibrillation
Heart failure with mildly reduced ejection fraction (HFmrEF; EF 45–49%)
History of high alcohol use—hepatic cirrhosis
Anxiety and depression
COPD

Medication

Beclometasone 100 mcg/dose inhaler od	Codeine 15 mg qds
Eplerenone 25 mg od	Ferrous fumarate 210 mg bd
Furosemide 40 mg od	Isosorbide mononitrate 40 mg bd
Omeprazole 10 mg od	Salbutamol 100 mcg/dose inhaler as required
Senna 15 mg at night	Sertraline 100 mg od
Tamsulosin 400 mcg MR od	Thiamine 100 mg bd
Trimethoprim 100 mg od long-term for UTI prevention	Paracetamol 1 g qds

DOI: 10.1201/9781003582007-8

Social History

Gordon lives in a care home that provides specialist dementia care. He is independently mobile and only intermittently uses a walking stick. He requires some assistance for most aspects of self-care. His family described him as able to hold conversations, which sometimes make sense but sometimes don't. His personality can be jovial or difficult. He is sometimes inappropriate in behaviour and conversation and resides in a male-only area of his care home for this reason. Recently, he hasn't been walking or socialising much and spends most of his time alone in his room. His family takes him in a wheelchair when they go out together. He hasn't drunk any alcohol or smoked any cigarettes since his heart attack and subsequent move into the care home 18 months ago.

Examination

He has normal alertness. His pulse is irregular, heart sounds are normal, and there is no peripheral oedema. Chest is clear. Abdomen is soft and non-tender with a urinary catheter in situ. His right leg is externally rotated, and he reports pain on any attempted movement. His leg pulses are present.

Six-Item Screener 1/6

4AT 3/12

BP 124/70 mmHg, pulse 84 bpm, oxygen saturation 94% on air, temperature 37.1°C, glucose 6.6 mmol/L, weight 68.0 kg

Investigations

Biochemistry	Value	Reference range	Haematology	Value	Reference range
Sodium	138	133–146 mmol/L	Haemoglobin	136	130–180 g/L
Potassium	4.6	3.5–5.3 mmol/L	MCV	95	82–100 fL
Urea	9.5	2.5–7.8 mmol/L	White cell count	8.7	4–11 10^9/L
Creatinine	110	64–104 umol/L	Platelets	258	140–400 10^9/L
C-reactive protein	36	< 5 mg/L			
Creatine kinase	956	25–200 U/L	Ferritin	48.0	12–250 ug/L

Liver blood tests, albumin, and calcium all normal

Urea 5.7 and creatinine 82 when taken six months ago

ECG—atrial fibrillation 79 bpm, right bundle branch block (also present on previous ECG)

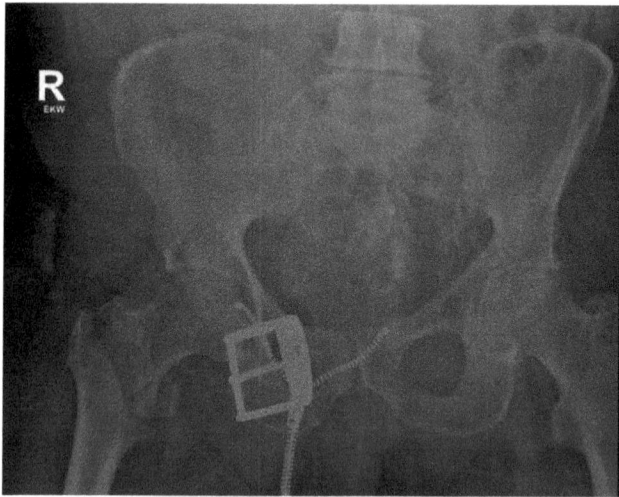

Figure 8.1 Pelvic X-ray showing a right intertrochanteric hip fracture.

Progress

Gordon was initially admitted under the orthopaedic team and had surgical fixation of his right hip fracture. A day later, he was transferred to the rehabilitation ward.

How would you reduce his future risk of recurrent hip fracture?
What is rehabilitation?

Reducing Future Fracture Risk

Gordon's hip fracture was caused by a fall. Reducing his risk of falling would reduce his risk of future fractures. He is at increased risk of falling because of cognitive impairment. He may forget his degree of functional limitation and not use the optimal mobility aid or try to get up without appropriate assistance. Prior to the fall, there were no features suggesting an acute illness. But he had no oedema detected on examination, and his blood tests showed his urea had risen, suggesting dehydration. Initially withholding his diuretics (furosemide and eplerenone) would be appropriate, with clinical review of the effect and repeat blood tests.

Orthostatic hypotension (OH) is common among older people and can contribute to risk of falling. A lying and standing blood pressure measurement may be able to detect this. Dehydration increases the risk of OH, as can many medications [see Case 11]. He is prescribed a large dose of isosorbide mononitrate. Now that he is less mobile, he may no longer get angina. It would be worth asking Gordon and those who know him well. A trial of dose reduction could be considered. Tamsulosin can also cause OH. Now that he has a long-term catheter, this can be discontinued. Sertraline can have mild anticholinergic effects and contribute to OH. The evidence for efficacy of antidepressants for people with dementia is also lacking [see Case 11]. An initial dose reduction to 50 mg daily is another option to discuss. Codeine, like other opiates, can increase the risk of falling. He may need an increase in analgesia around the time of his hip fracture, but this could be something to address in the future.

Gordon may also have underling osteoporosis that increased his risk of fracture with the fall. Medication may be able to strengthen his bones. Doing a DEXA scan to assess Gordon's bone density is a possibility. There is some evidence that zoledronate may reduce fracture risk in people following a hip fracture irrespective of bone density.[1] In a group of people with mean age 74, around 20 people needed to receive an annual intravenous zoledronate infusion for around two years to prevent one clinical fracture compared to placebo infusions. A potential adverse effect of a zoledronate infusion is a viral-like reaction with pyrexia, myalgia, and arthralgia lasting a few days. This could delay recovery and discharge for a vulnerable person like Gordon. Weighing up the potential risks and benefits includes estimating his life expectancy. Around 39% of people with dementia die in the year following a hip fracture.[2] Gordon has multi-morbidity and recent functional decline that both suggest his prognosis is worse than average.[3] Bisphosphonates take around a year to have a significant fracture-reducing effect. These data can help inform the shared decision-making process.

Rehabilitation

Rehabilitation aims to reduce the functional impact of deficits in physical or cognitive ability. Sometimes this is achieved through complete recovery from an illness. Sometimes residual deficits persist, and there is a need to adapt the way of performing tasks or by using specialised equipment.

A period of illness often results in temporarily reduced mobility. Being immobile promotes muscle loss. A study that assessed activity of previously mobile older people while in hospital found that, on average, 83% of their time was spent lying in bed, 13% sitting in chair, and just 4% standing up or walking around.[4] Even a small amount of muscle loss can have a significant functional impact on someone with frailty and sarcopenia. Trying to prevent muscle loss and deconditioning during a hospital admission is the ethos behind campaigns such as '#EndPJparalysis'.[5] This can also help avoid other sequelae of reduced mobility, including pressure ulcers and pneumonia. Patients should be encouraged to get out of bed and get dressed in normal clothes during the day as soon as possible during a hospital admission. This should be part of ward culture. Relatives or friends might be asked to bring in clean clothes.

There is a danger that mobilisation can be seen as something only done by physiotherapists. On a busy medical ward, physiotherapy input may be just 15 to 30 minutes per day per patient. This is unlikely to have a significant effect on muscle strength if the techniques are not utilised by other team members. For example, encourage people to be helped to mobilise to the toilet rather than rely on things that may seem more convenient in the short term, such as use of a bedpan.

Rehabilitation must be viewed as everyone's business. It is not a specific building and is better considered a mindset. It should occur in all areas of healthcare delivery. No one should wait for rehabilitation. It should start as early as possible in an acute admission with the aim of preventing deconditioning. Rehabilitation isn't just about mobility but more widely enabling people to be more independent. Incorporating small steps into routine practice helps achieve this goal, for example, ensuring the patient's call buzzer is in reach, a glass of water is available, and restrictive interventions are minimised (e.g. urinary catheter removed). The medical role in the rehab team is to optimise health and to anticipate any problems that may become barriers to improvement, such as pain, malnutrition/dehydration, poor sleep, depression, sensory barriers (e.g. visual/hearing impairment), physical barriers (e.g. OH), and bladder/bowel problems. If recovery isn't progressing as expected, has a problem been overlooked? Another role of the doctor can be to honestly predict the person's health trajectory. If there has been an inexorable decline in physical and cognitive function over several months due to an incurable disease (e.g. metastatic cancer, end-stage COPD, dementia), return to how things were six months ago is not realistic. Supporting the person/family/rehab team to understand this allows personalised decisions about what is important and can avoid unnecessary time away from home.

In older people, some functional decline can also occur outside of an acute illness episode. Advanced biological ageing eventually leads to organ impairment that affects ability to perform daily tasks. This is slowly progressive over months to years. People with frailty often have a rapid drop in function caused by an acute illness. The recovery from this is slower than for people without frailty, and they are at risk of some persisting functional loss, even when the acute condition has been fully treated.[6] There is a balance to be found between not giving sufficient rehabilitation input to optimise recovery and continuing to attempt rehabilitation when no further benefit will be obtained. Thinking about an individual's trajectory can help. Has this illness occurred after a period of stability, or is it on the background of functional decline?[7] We should consider the past, present, and future.

Past	Present	Future
Function two weeks prior to this admission	Function right now	Likely functional recovery Care needs and discharge plan

Choosing the right time for discharge can be difficult. Hospital care involves a balance of risks and benefits [see Case 7]. Although the ideal goal would be complete recovery prior to hospital discharge, this is not always possible, and sometimes getting home sooner is more important to the individual. Keeping someone in hospital because they are not 'back to baseline' can be unhelpful. Community rehabilitation teams may be able to continue within a patient's own home. The psychological impact of long stays in hospital for rehab can be to institutionalise the person making return to independence less likely, so the window for return home can be quite narrow and should not be missed.

Recovery from delirium can also be prolonged in older people with frailty, with some cognitive impairment frequently lasting for months.[8] People with pre-existing cognitive disorders are at greater risk. Episodes of delirium can lead to permanent deficits and greater risk of developing dementia. Although further improvement can occur once people are back in their more familiar home environment and routines.

What about Gordon?

Gordon required surgery to repair his broken hip and is then likely to need a period of rehabilitation. Prior to this admission, he had moderate frailty (CFS 6). Even with optimal treatment, his care needs may be increased at the time of discharge from hospital. We will need to ensure that his current care home can meet his future needs. Gordon's son already has Lasting Power of Attorney for his father's financial and health affairs. A 'do not attempt resuscitation order' was in place. He also had an emergency healthcare plan to avoid future hospital admission in most circumstances.

We have already talked about medications that could increase his risk of falling. It is also worth considering whether his other medicines are optimal for him. He is prescribed low-dose trimethoprim for long-term urinary tract infection (UTI) prevention. His long-term catheter will inevitably become colonised with bacteria, but there is little evidence to suggest that antibiotics can reduce the incidence of symptomatic UTI in someone like Gordon.[9] Instead, the bacteria colonising his catheter are likely to be resistant to common antibiotics, like trimethoprim, which could make any future UTI harder to treat. He is prescribed oral iron tablets for iron-deficiency anaemia. When this problem developed a year ago, it was agreed that Gordon would not tolerate investigations such as gastrointestinal endoscopy. The anticoagulant he was taking for atrial fibrillation was discontinued. The oral iron and a low dose of omeprazole have controlled this problem. The dose of iron that he is prescribed is higher than necessary, which may have adverse effects, e.g. constipation. A single tablet every other day is likely to be better tolerated.[10] Gordon had been started on thiamine supplementation several years ago when he had a high alcohol intake. He hasn't drunk any alcohol since moving into a care home. This medication can now be deprescribed. His inhaler technique should be checked, and the long-term balance of risks and benefit from his steroid inhaler should be reviewed [see Case 22].

Key Points

- Addressing risk factors for falling and considering bone health can reduce the future probability of fractures.
- Optimising medications for an individual can reduce falls risk and is an important aspect of CGA.
- Rehabilitation is not a building; it is everyone's business and should start soon after hospital admission to prevent deconditioning.
- Despite optimal care, some older people will have a new persisting functional deficit at the time of hospital discharge. This is also sometimes true for delirium.
- Think about past, present, and likely future function when considering illness trajectory and discharge planning.
- Work closely with therapists to ensure anything hindering improvement can be addressed early. Were your diagnoses correct? Has the treatment worked? Have they become confused/depressed?

Further Reading

1. Lyles KW, Colón-Emeric CS, Magaziner JS, et al. Zoledronic acid in reducing clinical fracture and mortality after hip fracture. *N Engl J Med* 2007;357:nihpa40967. https://doi.org/10.1056/NEJMoa074941

2. Bai J, Zhang P, Liang X, et al. Association between dementia and mortality in the elderly patients undergoing hip fracture surgery: a meta-analysis. *J Orthopedic Surg Res* 2018;13:298. https://doi.org/10.1186/s13018-018-0988-6

3. www.spict.org.uk

4. Brown CJ, Redden DT, Flood KL, et al. The underrecognized epidemic of low mobility during hospitalization of older adults. *J Am Geriatr Soc* 2009;57:1660–5. https://doi.org/10.1111/j.1532–5415.2009.02393.x

5. https://endpjparalysis.org/

6. Clegg A, Young J, Iliffe S, et al. Frailty in elderly people. *Lancet* 2013;381:752–62. https://doi.org/10.1016/S0140–6736(12)62167–9

7. Murray SA, Boyd K, Moine S, et al. Using illness trajectories to inform person centred, advance care planning. *BMJ* 2024;384:e067896. https://doi.org/10.1136/bmj-2021–067896

8. Cole MG, Bailey R, Bonnycastle M, et al. Partial and no recovery from delirium in older hospitalized adults: frequency and baseline risk factors. *J Am Geriatr Soc* 2015;63:2340–8. https://doi.org/10.1111/jgs.13791

9. Ahmed H, Davies F, Francis N, et al. Long-term antibiotics for prevention of recurrent urinary tract infection in older adults: systematic review and meta-analysis of randomised trials. *BMJ Open* 2017;7:e015233. https://doi.org/10.1136/bmjopen-2016–015233

10. Rimon E, Kagansky N, Kagansky M, et al. Are we giving too much iron? Low-dose iron therapy is effective in octogenarians. *Am J Med* 2005;118:1142–7. https://doi.org/10.1016/j.amjmed.2005.01.065

Case 9

Gloria

Gloria is an 82-year-old woman who presented to hospital with acute confusion. Recently, the district nursing team has been attending her home to change dressings on a venous ulcer on her legs. Two days ago, there was concern that she may have an infection developing around the ulcer over her left lateral malleolus. The district nurse contacted her GP, who prescribed antibiotics, but Gloria had only taken one dose before she came to hospital. In the morning, the district nurse visited again and found her on the floor and unable to get up. She had been incontinent of urine and appeared confused. Her blood glucose was recorded as 3.9 mmol/L by the ambulance crew in her home. She does not have a diagnosis of diabetes. She was given oral glucose gel by the paramedic.

In hospital, Gloria couldn't recall how she had fallen or for how long she had been stuck on the floor. She said that her legs have been 'bad' for a while. Her left leg is always worse than the right one. She had been feeling feverish the last few days. She had not had any nausea or vomiting. She had pain in her left leg. There was no chest or abdominal pain, breathlessness, nor recent viral type symptoms.

Past Medical History

Chronic kidney disease
Recurrent falls
Orthostatic hypotension (OH)
Previous cerebral infarct—13 years ago
Chronic venous leg ulcers
Vitamin B_{12} deficiency
Iron-deficiency anaemia—she declined gastrointestinal (GI) investigations a year ago

Medication

Amitriptyline 10 mg n	Atorvastatin 20 mg od
Betahistine 16 mg tds	Clopidogrel 75 mg od
Ferrous sulfate 200 mg od	Furosemide 20 mg od
Lansoprazole 15 mg od	Oxybutynin 5 mg bd
Oxycodone liquid 5 mg qds	Paracetamol 500 mg qds
Senna 15 mg od	Vitamin B_{12} injections three-monthly

DOI: 10.1201/9781003582007-9

Social History

Gloria lives alone in a bungalow and is mostly housebound. She is independent with activities of daily living. She usually furniture walks around her property. She uses a four-wheeled walking frame when she does go outdoors. She does not have any family who live locally. Her neighbour helps her with shopping.

Examination

Gloria has normal alertness. Irregular pulse, heart sounds normal. Chest clear. Abdomen soft and non-tender. Redness of left lower leg spreading to thigh. Left leg hot to touch and swollen compared to the right leg, with some pitting oedema. Right leg looks normal.

Six-Item Screener 2/6

4AT 7/12

BP 137/71 mmHg, pulse 115 bpm, oxygen saturation 93% on air, temperature 37.3°C

Investigations

Biochemistry	Value	Reference range	Haematology	Value	Reference range
Sodium	136	133–146 mmol/L	Haemoglobin	128	115–165 g/L
Potassium	4.8	3.5–5.3 mmol/L	MCV	80	82–100 fL
Urea	17.9	2.5–7.8 mmol/L	White cell count	15.4	4–11 10^9/L
Creatinine	155	49–90 umol/L	Neutrophils	14.6	2–7.5 10^9/L
C-reactive protein	265	< 5 mg/L	Platelets	161	140–400 10^9/L
			Ferritin	41	12–250 ug/L

Urea 8.5 and creatinine 96 one month ago, haemoglobin 112, MCV 75, and ferritin 13 a year ago
Viral swab for influenza/COVID was negative.
ECG—atrial fibrillation, 98 beats per minute

Why has Gloria developed delirium?
Why has she fallen over?
Would she benefit from anticoagulation for atrial fibrillation?

Delirium

Delirium is the term for acute cognitive impairment precipitated by exposure to a stressor. A range of risk factors increase susceptibility to developing delirium (see Table 9.1). Any acute illness could potentially make a person delirious. Only a minor stressor could precipitate delirium in a more vulnerable person, for example, a viral illness, new medication, or constipation. Whereas a major illness, such as sepsis, might be required to precipitate

Table 9.1 Delirium Risk Factors and Common Precipitants

Risk factors	Precipitants
Old age Pre-existing cognitive impairment Co-morbidities Polypharmacy Frailty Sensory impairment High alcohol intake	U—urinary retention/catheterisation P—pain I—infection N—nutritional problems C—constipation H—(de)hydration M—medications E—environment, e.g. unfamiliar, noisy

Table 9.2 Anticholinergic Burden—Typical Scores for More Commonly Prescribed Medications

Score 1 (mild)	Score 2 (moderate)	Score 3 (severe)

Antidepressants (except
    paroxetine and tricyclics)
Benzodiazepines
Digoxin
Furosemide
Haloperidol/risperidone
Metoclopramide
Opiates (except tramadol)
Steroids
	Amantadine
	Baclofen
	Cetirizine/loratadine
	Cimetidine/ranitidine
	Olanzapine/quetiapine
	Paroxetine
	Prochlorperazine
	Tramadol
		Bladder anticholinergics
		Chlorpheniramine/
		    hydroxyzine
		Clozapine
		Orphenadrine/procyclidine
		Tricyclic antidepressants

delirium in a more robust person. The mnemonic 'U PINCH ME' can help to search for common precipitants.

Gloria is vulnerable to delirium due to her degree of frailty, prior stroke, and combination of medications with anticholinergic effects. Various medications have anticholinergic properties, and this effect is amplified when taken in combination. Several scoring systems for anticholinergic effect have been developed. Although there is much overlap, scores for some medications vary between scales. Anticholinergic burden can be calculated by adding the relevant score for each medication (see Table 9.2). Long-term exposure to a high anticholinergic burden approximately doubles the risk of developing dementia.[1] On this occasion for Gloria, the precipitant has been development of left leg cellulitis.

The key steps in management are identifying and treating the trigger, i.e. antibiotics for Gloria's cellulitis, and trying to optimise risk factors. For Gloria, reducing medications with anticholinergic effects is a component of this. Anticholinergic medications can also increase the risk of falls either through cognitive impairment or potentiating OH [see Case 11]. Oxybutynin could be withheld. This type of medication has only limited evidence of efficacy, and an alternative approach to urinary symptoms is likely to be more appropriate for her [see Case 13]. Amitriptyline could also be withheld. She is only on a low dose so unlikely to experience withdrawal effects. At an appropriate time, it can be established why she is prescribed this medication and if she feels it has helped. An alternative approach may be more suitable. Beyond anticholinergic medications, opiates or anything that causes sedation can also precipitate delirium. Gloria is prescribed oxycodone. There is a balance to be found. Although this medication makes her more vulnerable to delirium, being in pain is also a trigger for delirium and not acceptable for her. Depending on symptom control, reducing the dose or switching to an alternative opiate medication or formulation (e.g. modified release) could be tried.

Fall

The causes of falls are outlined in Case 4. For Gloria, she has an acute illness that has led to delirium. Cognitive impairment affects judgment and recollection of own ability, e.g. requirement to use a walking aid. Subsequent dehydration and hypoglycaemia may also have played a role. In addition, she has OH, which is provoked by her combination of medications and current dehydration. A lying and standing blood pressure was performed. Her blood pressure fell from 134/59 mmHg to 97/67 mmHg a minute after standing. Treating the acute illness, rehydration, and limiting risk-increasing medications are key steps. Conveniently, this is very similar to the way we manage her delirium.

Anticoagulation for Atrial Fibrillation

Atrial fibrillation (AF) becomes more common as we get older, affecting around 10–20% of people aged over 80. The major risk is embolisation of clot formed within the cardiac atria to the brain, resulting in ischaemic stroke. Anticoagulant medication can reduce the relative risk of ischaemic stroke by around 60%. The absolute benefit depends on individual stroke risk, which can be estimated with the CHA_2DS_2-VA score. The CHA_2DS_2-VA score (range 0–8) is calculated from the following factors: congestive heart failure (1 point), hypertension (1 point), age $\geq$ 75 years (2 points), diabetes (1 point), history of stroke or TIA (2 points), other vascular disease (1 point), and age 65–74 years (1 point). Table 9.3 shows the approximate annual risk of stroke for people at various scores and the effect size of benefit from anticoagulation.[2]

Direct oral anticoagulants (DOAC; e.g. apixaban, edoxaban, rivaroxaban) are easier to take than the older drug warfarin (i.e. no monitoring), offer the same reduction in thromboembolism risk, and have a lower risk of bleeding complications. With DOAC, the

Table 9.3 CHA_2DS_2-VA Score and Benefit of Anticoagulation by Number Need to Treat (NNT) per Year to Prevent One Stroke [Based on Reference 2]

CHA_2DS_2-VA score	Stroke risk per year	NNT per year
0	0.5	333
1	1.2	139
2	2.6	64
3	5.0	33
4	8.0	21
5	12.1	14
6 to 8	18.1	9

risk of major bleeding is 1.6–3.6% per year and intracranial haemorrhage is 0.2–0.5% per year.[3] At very low ischaemic stroke risk, the adverse effects of anticoagulation are likely to exceed the beneficial effects. Current guidelines recommend offering anticoagulation to people with a CHA_2DS_2-VA score of 2 or more.[4]

The benefit of anticoagulation may become attenuated in very old people with moderate to severe frailty due to a greater risk of medication adverse effects and limited life expectancy. Bleeding risk scores (e.g. ORBIT) are not recommended to guide prescribing.[4] An analysis suggests that, on average, beyond the age of 92, a net benefit may be lost for DOAC medications for preventing stroke with AF.[5] Of course, these data don't mean that nobody benefits from anticoagulation beyond this age but do suggest a more cautious approach is needed for people with a greater degree of frailty. Another factor affecting risk is cognition. Data suggest the risk of serious adverse effects with anticoagulation is doubled in people with cognitive impairment.[6] This may be partly explained by an association with cerebral amyloid angiopathy [see Case 24]. Another factor that would go against a decision to anticoagulate is a history of major bleeding, such as an intracranial bleed, unless an underlying source has been identified and treated.

Gloria's CHA_2DS_2-VA score is 4. Currently, she is acutely unwell. It is possible that the AF could resolve when she recovers. We could repeat her ECG or do a prolonged ambulatory ECG. Given she has delirium, we can postpone the anticoagulation decision to allow her to recover and then be involved in the decision-making process. Another issue for Gloria is iron-deficiency anaemia. She had declined GI investigations in the past and was commenced on low-dose iron and a proton pump inhibitor, in addition to remaining on clopidogrel to reduce future stroke risk. Clopidogrel doesn't reduce stroke risk in AF, so it could now be stopped. Certainly, she should not be co-prescribed antiplatelet and anticoagulant medications. There is no easy right or wrong answer here, hence, the need to get Gloria's input. If she recovers well from her cellulitis, then she may wish to reconsider GI investigations prior to anticoagulation. What is the most important goal for her, i.e. avoiding a thromboembolic stroke or avoiding a major bleed?

What about Gloria?

Gloria has mild frailty (CFS 5). She was treated with an antibiotic, initially intravenously, for her cellulitis. She also had initial intravenous fluids for dehydration, and furosemide was discontinued. Her medicines were optimised. The low blood sugar was probably just due to reduced oral intake because she was unwell and immobile. Subsequent values were within the normal range. Her delirium improved, and she had no further falls. After discussing the risks and benefits, she decided to commence apixaban to reduce risk of stroke, and her clopidogrel was stopped. She did not want to have GI investigations to try to find the source of her iron deficiency.

Why does Goria take betahistine? Dizziness is a vague term that is sometimes used to describe light-headedness, vertigo, or an imbalance sensation. Try to clarify which of these is occurring to help identify the cause of the symptom. Betahistine is a medication that is sometimes prescribed for vertigo symptoms caused by a vestibular system impairment. It probably works via histamine H3 receptor antagonism and has weak evidence of some benefit.[7] Short-term use with an acute disorder, such as vestibular neuritis, might be considered, but it may not have any long-term benefit for chronic conditions.

Light-headedness related to postural change is most likely to be caused by orthostatic hypotension. A chronic imbalance sensation could be caused by cerebrovascular disease for Gloria.[8] These latter two conditions will not be improved by betahistine use. A trial without is a reasonable option to discuss.

Key Points

- Relatively minor insults can provoke delirium in susceptible people.
- Anticholinergic drug exposure increases the risk of cognitive decline.
- Taking several medications with anticholinergic properties amplifies this risk.
- CHA_2DS_2-VA score can be used to estimate the potential benefit of anticoagulation for an individual with AF.
- Limited life expectancy, severe frailty, and cognitive impairment can attenuate the benefit of anticoagulation for AF to prevent stroke.

Further Reading

1. Taylor-Rowan M, Edwards S, Noel-Storr AH, et al. Anticholinergic burden (prognostic factor) for prediction of dementia or cognitive decline in older adults with no known cognitive syndrome. *Cochrane Database Syst Rev* 2021;Issue 5. Art. No.: CD013540. https://doi.org/10.1002/14651858.CD013540.pub2
2. Teppo K, Lip GYH, Airaksinen EJ, et al. Comparing CHA2DS2-VA and CHA2DS2-VASc scores for stroke risk stratification in patients with atrial fibrillation: a temporal trends analysis from the retrospective Finnish AntiCoagulation in Atrial Fibrillation (FinACAF) cohort. *Lancet Regional Health Europe* 2024;43:100967. https://doi.org/10.1016/j.lanepe.2024.100967
3. Eikelboom J, Merli G. Bleeding with direct oral anticoagulants vs warfarin: clinical experience. *Am J Med* 2016;129:S33–S40. https://doi.org/10.1016/j.amjmed.2016.06.003
4. European Society of Cardiology. 2024 ESC Guidelines for the management of atrial fibrillation developed in collaboration with the European Association for Cardio-Thoracic Surgery (EACTS). *Eur Heart J* 2024;45:3314–414. https://doi.org/10.1093/eurheartj/ehae176
5. Shah SJ, Singer DE, Fang MC, et al. Net clinical benefit of oral anticoagulation among older adults with atrial fibrillation. *Circ Cardiovasc Qual Outcomes* 2019;12:e006212. https://doi.org/10.1161/CIRCOUTCOMES.119.006212
6. Wang W, Lessard D, Kiefe CI, et al. Differential effect of anticoagulation according to cognitive function and frailty in older patients with atrial fibrillation. *J Am Geriatr Soc* 2023;71:394–403. https://doi.org/10.1111/jgs.18079
7. Murdin L, Hussain K, Schilder AGM. Betahistine for symptoms of vertigo. *Cochrane Database Syst Rev* 2016;Issue 6. Art. No.: CD010696. https://doi.org/10.1002/14651858.CD010696.pub2
8. Ibitoye RT, Castro P, Cooke J, et al. A link between frontal white matter integrity and dizziness in cerebral small vessel disease. *NeuroImage: Clinical* 2022;35:103098. https://doi.org/10.1016/j.nicl.2022.103098

Gladys

Gladys is an 88-year-old woman who was brought to the hospital following a fall at home. She was seen by the emergency department doctor along with her daughter, Clare. Gladys couldn't recall events around the fall. Clare had found her in the bathroom on the floor unable to get up. Her mother didn't appear hurt or have any sign of having banged her head. Gladys had been increasingly confused over the preceding week, and she had not been eating or drinking well. Clare phoned their GP, who was also concerned about the deterioration, and had come to visit her more than once. Gladys had only been passing small volumes of urine recently but passed a normal bowel motion two days prior to her fall. She had been more breathless on mobilising, and her GP had prescribed a course of steroids, for a possible COPD exacerbation, but her daughter had not yet given her any because she was worried about adverse effects to her stomach while not eating.

Past Medical History

COPD
Type 2 diabetes (retinopathy)
Ischaemic heart disease (myocardial infarction seven years ago)

Mixed dementia—Gladys's cognition seemed to rapidly decline three years ago when her partner died and deteriorated further after the death of her son from alcoholism one year ago.

Medication

Alogliptin 25 mg od	Aspirin 75 mg od
Bisoprolol 2.5 mg od	Cyanocobalamin 50 mcg od
Furosemide 40 mg od	Losartan 100 mg od
Metformin 500 mg bd	

Social History

Gladys is a retired English teacher, and her main passion was reading novels, but this stopped due to her declining eyesight and memory. Since the death of her partner, she lives alone in an upstairs flat. She can mobilise short distances using a wheeled walking frame with minimal assistance. Carers attend three times a day, and Clare helps too. She needs some assistance with all her personal care. Her carers also prompt with medicine-taking from her multi-dose compartment box, but Gladys had frequently declined to take the tablets over the last few

DOI: 10.1201/9781003582007-10

weeks. There was a recent incident when she left the gas from the cooker on, but fortunately, no harm resulted. She is a current smoker. Clare feels that her mother is no longer safe at home alone and was staying with her overnight for the last week.

Examination

Gladys is drowsy but opens her eye to voice. Her pupils are equal and reactive to light. Power does not appear diminished and is symmetrical in her limbs. Cardio-respiratory and abdominal examination are normal, including no sign of oedema. Her skin appears in good condition, and there is no significant bruising. No signs of bone injury are detected.

4AT 10/12

Six-Item Screener 0/6

BP 127/56 mmHg, pulse 112 bpm, oxygen saturation 94% on air, temperature 36.5°C, weight 48.9 kg, glucose 9.0 mmol/L (in range 7 to 15 during admission)

Investigations

Biochemistry	Value	Reference range	Haematology	Value	Reference range
Sodium	128	133–146 mmol/L	Haemoglobin	136	115–165 g/L
Potassium	5.6	3.5–5.3 mmol/L	MCV	88	82–100 fL
Urea	7.4	2.5–7.8 mmol/L	White cell count	8.1	4–11 10^9/L
Creatinine	154	49–90 umol/L	Platelets	284	140–400
C-reactive protein	4	< 5 mg/L			10^9/L
Bicarbonate	15	22–29 mmol/L	Hb_{A1C}	104	20–42 mmol/mol
Magnesium	0.53	0.7–1.0 mmol/L			
TSH	1.4	0.3–4.5 mIU/L	Vitamin B_{12}	146	150–1000 ng/L
Cortisol (random)	542	140–690 nmol/L	Folate	3.4	1–18.8 ug/L
Serum osmolality	271	275–295 mosmol/kg	Ferritin	31	12–250 ug/L

Two weeks ago: sodium 129, potassium 4.5, urea 5.5, creatinine 95
Liver blood tests and calcium in normal range
Urine: osmolality 274 mosmol/kg, sodium 45 mmol/L, potassium 23 mmol/L
Chest X-ray—normal
CT head—atrophy and small vessel ischaemic changes, no acute lesion

What should we do about her blood test results?
How would you tackle her diabetes management now and in the future?
What is her life expectancy?
Would advance care planning be useful, and how might you explore it?

Abnormal Blood Tests

Gladys has hyponatraemia [also see Case 6], probably contributed to by diuretic medication and poorly controlled diabetes. Furosemide promotes renal sodium loss. Her high urinary sodium concentration is consistent with this. She has no current clinical evidence of fluid overload, and her urea is raised, suggesting mild dehydration. Angiotensin receptor antagonists, such as losartan, are occasionally associated with hyponatraemia. High potassium is probably due to the combination of losartan and dehydration. Stopping furosemide and losartan, getting her blood sugars under control, and giving oral fluids could start to tackle her hyponatraemia and hyperkalaemia. Giving intravenous fluids would be possible if the initial steps were insufficient. Due to delirium, she may not tolerate this well, and there is a risk of over-correcting her fluid deficit leading to overload. Acidosis (low bicarbonate) also leads to hyperkalaemia. Correcting this is another possible option, e.g. oral sodium bicarbonate tablets.

Low magnesium can be caused by diuretics, such as furosemide. Other medications, such as proton pump inhibitors, are sometimes implicated. Poor diabetic control could also have an effect. While low magnesium can cause symptoms, including delirium, her serum concentration is only mildly reduced and will probably correct with the other management steps. Intravenous replacement can be used for severe cases (e.g. symptomatic and/or < 0.4 mmol/L). Oral replacement tastes unpleasant and is often poorly tolerated. An initial goal is to restore her to eating and drinking sufficiently to survive. Reducing her medication burden could help achieve this aim.

Type 2 Diabetes Management

Type 2 diabetes (T2DM) management for older people with frailty and dementia has a different risk-benefit profile compared with other phases of life. The past ten years of glycaemic control determines the future ten-year risk of vascular complications. Given that Gladys's life expectancy is well below ten years, maintaining tight glycaemic control is unlikely to be very helpful for her. The key is to minimise both hypoglycaemic events and symptomatic hyperglycaemia (i.e. polydipsia, polyuria, dehydration, headaches, and weight loss).

The classic adrenergic symptoms of hypoglycaemia are sweating, tremor, and palpitations. These become less common in older people, and presentations with neurological symptoms are more common (e.g. slurred speech, ataxia, visual disturbances, falls, confusion, and seizures). Glucose is the brain's key energy source, yet it can't store or create it. Brain tissue is particularly vulnerable to hypoglycaemia, and severe episodes are associated with an increased risk of cognitive decline.[1] This is especially important to someone like Gladys, who already has a vulnerable brain. Reduced awareness of hypoglycaemia and variable eating patterns also increase the risk for people with dementia. Living alone also makes hypoglycaemia riskier. For people at high risk, like Gladys, a lenient blood glucose target is sensible. Aiming for an Hb_{A1C} within the range 64 to 75 mmol/mol lowers the risk of hypoglycaemia and is unlikely to lead to symptoms of hyperglycaemia. A range of therapeutic options are available to achieve this goal. Key characteristics of these are outlined in Table 10.1.

Gladys's most recent Hb_{A1C} was 104, suggesting poor control. She was no longer able to self-manage her diabetes and had not been taking her medications reliably for several weeks.

Table 10.1 Key Characteristics of Commonly Prescribed Classes of Medications for T2DM

Medication type	Effect on glucose	Risk of hypoglycaemia	Weight change	Notes
Insulin	High	High	Gain	
Metformin	Moderate	Low	Loss	Can cause vitamin B_{12} deficiency
Sulphonylureas	Moderate	High	Small gain	
GLP-1 analogues	Moderate	Low	Large loss	
Pioglitazone	Low	Low	Little effect	Not for people with heart failure
DPP4 inhibitors	Low	Low	Little effect	
SGLT2 inhibitors	Low	Low	Small loss	Risk of volume depletion/falls, urinary tract infection

Hyperglycaemia exacerbates dehydration and hyponatraemia through osmotic effects. On admission, her blood glucose was not very elevated, but her oral intake had declined by that stage. While in hospital, we can monitor her blood glucose, but we must acknowledge that both her medication adherence and oral intake may be quite different once she returns home.

What we discovered for Gladys was that despite her metformin being initially withheld due to dehydration and acidosis, her blood sugar was reasonably controlled on her usual alogliptin alone. This indicated that the primary need was to support her in balancing her oral intake and medication. Reducing the complexity of her prescription by deprescribing made this easier. The food she received in hospital may be very different from what she eats at home, and her appetite may be reduced due to acute illness. This would need to be monitored in the future.

Metformin can impair vitamin B_{12} absorption, leading to deficiency. Gladys had been prescribed cyanocobalamin supplementation for this reason. Metformin also commonly causes gastrointestinal side effects, reduced appetite, and weight loss. Given Gladys's reduced oral intake and low body mass, this is not helpful for her. While Gladys's vitamin B_{12} was low, her haemoglobin and MCV were normal, and it was reasonable to see how this changed off metformin. Control of T2DM is easier when weight declines, which is a common feature of frailty. Previously required medications can sometimes be reduced or discontinued.

What is Gladys's Life Expectancy?

Acknowledging that there is a risk of deterioration and death when a frail older person is ill in hospital is often valuable because it allows people to prepare and consider options open to them.

Nobody knows exactly what the future holds, and we can't predict life expectancy to the hour or minute, but we can use available information to provide some guidance. Life expectancy data give average survivals for people at any given age. In the UK, a woman aged 88, on average, will live to age 94 or for six more years.[2] It can be easy to forget that older people in hospital are just a small section of older people. Gladys isn't an average woman aged 88. She has multiple co-morbidities and has presented to hospital with an acute health crisis. She has severe frailty (CFS 7), requiring assistance with all personal care, due to a combination of physical and cognitive impairments. For people over 85 years of age, average mortality approaches 50% in the year after an admission.[3] The Supportive and Palliative Care Indicators Tool is an example of a resource that can help to identify people with reduced life expectancy.[4] Considering all the available information, Gladys is likely to be within her last year of life.

Advance Care Planning Including 'Do Not Resuscitate'

Agreeing the general approach to health problems, or the 'philosophy of care', involves discussion about preventative, curative, disease modifying, symptomatic, and palliative types of treatments. These are not mutually exclusive (i.e. the healthcare professional should always look to alleviate suffering while considering diagnostic and treatment plans) and are not static over time (e.g. initial attempts to cure an infection may turn to a purely palliative approach as multi-organ failure sets in). In medicine, we can't predict the future with accuracy. Some people will benefit from treatments we offer; others will develop adverse effects. Shared decision-making promotes patient involvement in choices about their healthcare to ensure they align with their own goals and values.[5] We should ask: What matters to you? The following are examples of the type of response we could receive:

- 'I just want to make it to November because my niece is getting married'.
- 'I would rather die than end up in a care home not knowing who I was'.
- 'I'll try anything. I have to get better because my wife needs me'.

These need further exploration, but they certainly help us understand the person's perspective. If you can reach an agreement as to what the realistic life goals are for your patient in the context of their current and long-term illnesses, it is much easier to discuss the potential benefits and risks of treatment plans. This includes the emotive 'resuscitation decision'. It is wise to attempt to have these conversations openly and honestly and at a time ahead of the crisis point wherever possible.

Despite advances in medical treatments, resuscitation after in-hospital cardiac arrest does not have a high chance of survival to discharge and has an even lower chance of getting back to prior function. The treatment is invasive and very physical. Remember that deteriorating health despite optimal interventions is an indication of impending death. When organ failure leads to the heart stopping beating, chest compressions and cardioversion aren't an effective treatment. This is not the same as the original paradigm of cardiac arrest where a primary cardiac rhythm problem stops cardiac output.

Data from the UK suggest that around 11% of people aged 80 and over survive to discharge following in-hospital cardiac arrest.[6] However, analysing data by frailty status shows that this has a major influence. In two UK studies, just 0 to 2% of people with CFS score > 5 survived.[7,8] Modern post-arrest care routinely involves time in a critical care environment for invasive monitoring and treatment. Return of spontaneous circulation is, therefore, the beginning of a long journey to recovery, which entails more treatments, attempts at treating the causal illness, and a period of rehabilitation during which the person remains vulnerable to further insults. Reduced cerebral perfusion risks hypoxic brain injury, resulting in persisting physical or cognitive functional impairment. Limited data suggest that 30 to 50% of cardiac arrest survivors have some persisting cognitive impairment.[9] For people with frailty, it can be useful to understand that following cardiopulmonary resuscitation, by far the most likely outcome is death, then a small chance of surviving in a more disabled state, and then a very small chance of surviving to independence.

When people lack capacity to engage in this complex and abstract conversation, seeking advocacy is a vital part of understanding best interest [see Case 6]. It is not easy for family members to be involved in these discussions, however, as they often feel they are giving up on their loved one if they agree with a 'do not resuscitate' form. It can be much more useful to clarify what they think the person themselves would think or want given the current situation and build the escalation plan around increasing the chance of achieving that.

Because of Gladys's cognitive impairment, she lacked mental capacity to discuss resuscitation. Her daughter, Clare, as next of kin, was included in the conversation. Based on the low probability of a survival to independence and Gladys's long-held view that she would not want to survive in a disabled state in a care home, a decision was made that completing a 'do not resuscitate' form was in her best interests. It was made very clear to Gladys and Clare that this would not prevent her getting all the other medical treatments that could still benefit her.

What about Gladys?

Gladys had a very difficult time in the hospital. Although she initially improved, she suffered further acute illnesses, and when she did, her care needs had increased. With Clare's increasing support, Gladys had been able to continue living in her own home. Clare now recognised that her mother's health was failing and that she had recently been under increasing carer strain. She didn't feel she could carry on supporting her mother like this. By working with the multi-disciplinary team, a discharge plan was created.

On leaving the hospital, Gladys moved into a care home, dependent for all her activities of daily living and mobile with a two-wheeled walking frame plus assistance of one person. Given how difficult she had found the hospital environment and how she had continued to deteriorate with treatment, we discussed her ongoing healthcare plans with her daughter and GP and agreed that a more specific focus on symptom control should be adopted in the event of further acute health problems. This was about recognising that Gladys had been physically and cognitively declining quite rapidly and was entering the last phase of her life. Treatments aimed at cure were less likely to work and, if successful (at avoiding death), were more likely to leave her even more impaired. Treatment aimed at symptoms might allow her to enjoy time with family in comfort as she neared the end of her life. She continued to decline in the care home and died there a month later.

Key Points

- The goals of T2DM management in older people with frailty differ from younger, less frail people. Avoiding hypoglycaemia is more important that the prevention of long-term vascular complications.
- Estimating life expectancy can help inform discussions about care.

- Cardiorespiratory resuscitation has only very small chance of a successful outcome in older people with frailty and may lead to persisting physical or cognitive impairment.
- Shared decision-making can help to align treatment choices with individual goals and values.

Further Reading

1. Huang L, Zhu M, Ji J. Association between hypoglycemia and dementia in patients with diabetes: a systematic review and meta-analysis of 1.4 million patients. *Diabetol Metab Syndrome* 2022;14:31. https://doi.org/10.1186/s13098-022-00799-9

2. https://www.ons.gov.uk/peoplepopulationandcommunity/healthandsocialcare/healthandlifeexpectancies/articles/lifeexpectancycalculator/2019-06-07

3. Clark D, Armstrong M, Allan A, et al. Imminence of death among hospital inpatients: prevalent cohort study. *Palliative Med* 2014;28:474–9. https://doi.org/10.1177/0269216314526443

4. www.spict.org.uk

5. *NICE Shared Decision Making.* 2021. www.nice.org.uk/guidance/ng197

6. Nolan JP, Soar J, Smith GB, et al. Incidence and outcome of in-hospital cardiac arrest in the United Kingdom National Cardiac Arrest Audit. *Resuscitation* 2014;85:987–92. https://doi.org/10.1016/j.resuscitation.2014.04.002

7. Wharton C, King E, MacDuff A. Frailty is associated with adverse outcome from in-hospital cardiopulmonary resuscitation. *Resuscitation* 2019;143:208–11. https://doi.org/10.1016/j.resuscitation.2019.07.021

8. Ibitoye SE, Rawlinson S, Cavanagh A, et al. Frailty status predicts futility of cardiopulmonary resuscitation in older adults. *Age Ageing* 2021;50:147–52. https://doi.org/10.1093/ageing/afaa104

9. Green CR, Botha JA, Tiruvoipati R. Cognitive function, quality of life and mental health in survivors of out-of-hospital cardiac arrest: a review. *Anaesth Intensive Care* 2015;43:568–76. https://doi.org/10.1177/0310057X1504300504

Angela

Angela is a 94-year-old retired physiotherapist who was brought to hospital after a fall in her residential care home. Since the fall, the staff in her care home had seen her clutching her right shoulder, and she had not been walking around as usual. Angela had no recollection of falling. When asked about pain, she pointed to right shoulder. She did not describe any other painful locations. No nausea or vomiting had been noticed.

A collateral history was obtained from the staff at her care home. This fall had not been witnessed. A staff member had heard raised voices from down the corridor. When she arrived at the scene, Angela was lying on the floor. It was unclear if there had been an altercation with another care home resident or if Angela had simply lost her balance. Unfortunately, it took over an hour for the ambulance to arrive, and she remained on the floor for that time (the staff were worried they may cause her an injury if they tried to move her). Angela also had a fall four months ago, which resulted in a fractured clavicle, and she spent two weeks in hospital. Her mobility had returned to baseline after that admission, and she walks independently without using a mobility aid. There was no current illness outbreak in the care home. Angela had a good appetite, and no change had been noted in her bowels or passing urine. She has lost a few kilograms of weight over recent months.

Past Medical History

Dementia
Osteoporosis
Bilateral pulmonary emboli diagnosed two years ago
Fall with right clavicular fracture four months ago
Left greater trochanter fracture ten years ago
Glaucoma
Osteoarthritis

Medication

Apixaban 2.5 mg bd	Bimatoprost 300/timolol 5 eye drops both eyes od
Colecalciferol 800 units od	
Lansoprazole 15 mg od	Dorzolamide 20 mg/ml eye drops L eye bd
Paracetamol 500 mg as required	
Sertraline 100 mg od	Macrogol one sachet bd
	Senna 15 mg nocte as required

DOI: 10.1201/9781003582007-11

Social History

Angela lives in a residential care home that provides specialist dementia care. She requires assistance for all her personal care. She is independently mobile without a walking aid and can feed herself. Angela's only daughter visits her regularly. Angela has a very poor memory and often refers to her daughter as her sister, but she can express her needs. She has never smoked and has never been a regular drinker of alcohol.

Examination

Angela was alert, chatty, and in good spirits. She had some crackles at the left lung base, but otherwise, her cardiac, respiratory, and abdominal examination was normal. She was tender over the right acromioclavicular joint. She had full range of movement of the shoulder but with crepitus. She was tender at the right fourth metacarpophalangeal joint with bruising and swelling. Her hips moved ok without pain. There was nothing to suggest head injury, and neurological examination was unremarkable.

Six-Item Screener 2/6

Her initial observations were all normal, weight 42.0 kg.

Lying-standing blood pressure revealed a drop from 153/85 mmHg to 90/61 mmHg after one minute.

Investigations

Biochemistry	Value	Reference range	Haematology	Value	Reference range
Sodium	139	133–146 mmol/L	Haemoglobin	117	115–165 g/L
Potassium	3.8	3.5–5.3 mmol/L	MCV	78	82–100 fL
Urea	11.6	2.5–7.8 mmol/L	White cell count	10.9	4–11 10⁹/L
Creatinine	76	49–90 umol/L	Platelets	295	140–400 10⁹/L
C-reactive protein	48	< 5 mg/L			

Urea 8.7 and creatinine 74 six weeks ago
Shoulder and hand radiographs showed no new bony injury.
ECG—sinus rhythm, 83 bpm

Progress

Angela was started on oral antibiotics for a possible chest infection, based on the chest signs, pleural effusion, and raised C-reactive protein. She was also given analgesia and assessed by the physiotherapy team. Angela's family were worried about the multiple falls in her care home and whether she is getting the supervision that she needs. They wondered if communication between hospital and care home staff surrounding supervision and mobility needs is not clear enough, leading to her multiple falls.

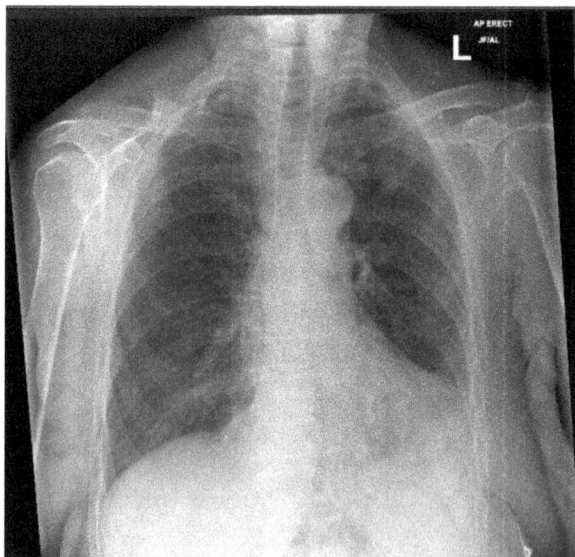

Figure 11.1 Chest X-ray showing a left basal pleural effusion, hyperexpanded lungs, and an old right clavicular fracture.

Does Angela have orthostatic hypotension, and what could we do about it?
Should she continue taking apixaban?
What should we do about her weight loss?
Is sertraline likely to have a net beneficial effect for Angela?

Orthostatic Hypotension

Orthostatic hypotension (OH) is defined as a 'sustained' drop in systolic blood pressure (BP) of 20 mmHg or diastolic blood pressure of 10 mmHg within three minutes of moving from lying to standing or a drop in BP to below 90 mmHg systolic. While some people describe classical symptoms (i.e. light-headedness, coat hanger pain, blurred vision), others use more subtle descriptions, and it can be just the postural element or a specific task that brings it on. For others, it is something a friend or relative notices (e.g. 'goes pale'). Impaired cerebral perfusion reduces cognitive function, balance, and truncal tone, which increases the risk of falling. In older people, it is more common with, and made worse by, medications that limit usual physiological responses of the cardiovascular system following change in posture. OH affects around 25% of people aged over 85 or who reside in a care home.[1] Potential ways to tackle OH fall into lifestyle adjustments (see Table 11.1), deprescribing, and physical measures (e.g. abdominal binder). Only if significant symptoms persist after these adjustments might medications to raise BP be considered.

Medications Causing Orthostatic Hypotension

Many medications can precipitate OH (see Figure 11.2). Medicine reduction is often key to the treatment of OH and falls in older people with multi-morbidity. It may be necessary to

Table 11.1 Lifestyle Measures that Can Reduce the Risk of Orthostatic Hypotension

Things to try	Things to avoid
Keep well hydrated Drink a full glass of water before getting up Smaller meals more often Take time when going from lying or sitting to standing Clench the hands and wriggle the feet before standing Sit or lie down if symptoms occur	Hot rooms Rapid or prolonged standing Very large meals Alcohol

Physiological changes on standing

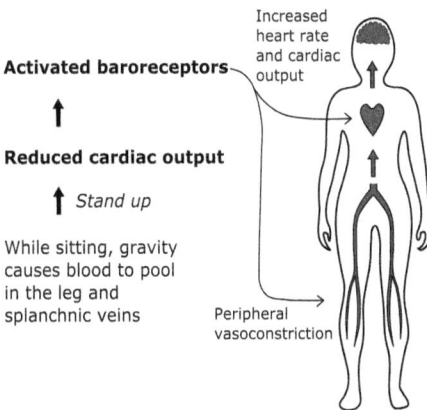

Medication effects

Increased heart rate and cardiac output

Activated baroreceptors

Reduced cardiac output

↑ *Stand up*

While sitting, gravity causes blood to pool in the leg and splanchnic veins

Peripheral vasoconstriction

Cardiac output
Heart rate: beta-blockers, diltiazem
Volume depletion: diuretics

Autonomic nervous system
Anti-cholinergics

Vasodilation
Alpha-blockers
Antihypertensives
Antianginals
Dopaminergics

Figure 11.2 Medications that can provoke orthostatic hypotension.

deprescribe medicines that are indicated for other health conditions if the person cannot get up and move around without falling because of OH. Older people with frailty who are immobile swiftly become deconditioned, lose muscle bulk, and risk related illnesses, such as pressure ulcers and pneumonia. This is a huge threat to independence and so people often choose to reduce the immediate risk of falls over other longer term health risk prevention. For people with supine hypertension, a more lenient BP target may be a practical trade-off. In the UK, NICE guidance for hypertension suggests measuring BP both while seated and one minute after standing for people with OH.[2] The lower value obtained should be used to guide therapeutic decisions.

Other Management Options

Compression garments, such as abdominal binders, might reduce OH symptoms by improving venous return to the heart. There is only weak evidence of benefit from clinical trials. They can be uncomfortable to wear, and patient acceptance/adherence tends to be low.

Fludrocortisone is a medicine sometimes prescribed for OH. It is a synthetic mineralocorticoid, working like aldosterone to retain sodium and water. Possible adverse effects include fluid retention and hypokalaemia. It is contraindicated for people with heart failure or prescribed diuretic medications. It has the potential to increase BP, but an ability to reduce episodes of falls or syncope has not been demonstrated in a clinical trial.

Midodrine is an alpha-agonist. Its action is to vasoconstrict arterioles, leading to a rise in BP. The evidence base for its use is mainly around autonomic failure and vasovagal syncope in young people, where it increases blood pressure and can reduce symptoms. The evidence for improving outcomes in older adults is very weak. The most serious potential adverse effects are related to supine hypertension. It is illogical to co-prescribe midodrine with any anti-hypertensive or vasodilating medications. Midodrine could induce urinary retention in men with prostatic enlargement, and it should not be co-prescribed with an alpha blocker, such as tamsulosin.

Should Angela Continue Anticoagulation?

For Angela, the potential benefit of anticoagulation with apixaban was to reduce the risk of recurrent pulmonary emboli, which could cause symptoms and even sudden death. The risks of bleeding had previously been identified, but the practical implication, such as being brought to hospital for urgent assessment each time she fell over, could become a significant burden.

Long-term anti-coagulation is often recommended for pulmonary emboli that occurred without an identified provoking factor. The reason for this is a relatively high risk of recurrence after treatment cessation, estimated around 10% in the first year off treatment, 16% over two years, 25% at five years, and 36% after ten years.[3] Anticoagulant treatment reduces the risk of recurrence by up to 90%, but this is partially offset by an increased risk of bleeding complications.[4] Major bleeding has an estimated risk around 1% per year for people taking a DOAC, like apixaban. However, risks may be higher in older people with frailty. One analysis suggested a doubling of risk for people with cognitive impairment.[5] These data don't give us a definitive right or wrong answer, but they can aid discussions in a shared decision-making process. Angela's cognitive impairment may mean she can't decide the best course of action for herself. Her daughter could be involved in discussions to establish what is in Angela's best interests.

Weight Loss

Angela has a small pleural effusion and has lost weight. It is possible that she has lung cancer, but she has never smoked. A follow-up chest X-ray six weeks after she has been treated for pneumonia, to ensure resolution, is the recommended practice. This is to identify whether further investigation is indicated to diagnose underlying lung cancer. For Angela, knowing that she had a lung cancer would not alter the available treatments and so the value would primarily have been for others to prognosticate and plan more easily. The burden is the visit to the hospital for an appointment at radiology services and any subsequent investigations and follow-up. There are many other possible explanations for her weight loss. Developing frailty is often associated with losing weight. Her oral intake may have declined because of dementia.

Appetite and the pleasurable sensations of eating can diminish. In the context of her limited life expectancy, an approach that prioritises symptom control is likely to be appropriate. Ensuring that she is offered the foods that she likes to eat and given optimal assistance may benefit her more than any imaging studies.

Antidepressant Medications for People with Dementia

Affective symptoms commonly occur in people with dementia. They include low mood, anxiety, and apathy. Unfortunately, standard antidepressant treatments have not been found to be effective and may only result in adverse effects.[6] Common adverse effects of selective serotonin reuptake inhibitors (SSRI) include nausea and constipation. Anticholinergic adverse effect can contribute to OH, falls risk, and cognitive impairment. SSRI tend to be less sedating than other types of antidepressants, such as mirtazapine. It is useful to consider the previous and current effectiveness of antidepressant medications when prescribed for someone with dementia who has fallen. For Angela, an initial reduction of sertraline dose to 50 mg od, followed by discontinuation after two weeks if there has been no adverse effect, is an option to discuss. This could reduce her risk of falling due to OH and could possibly have a small benefit for cognition.

What about Angela?

Angela has severe frailty (CFS 7). Her family had seen her deteriorating recently with more falls and worsening mobility. She had lost weight, and her dementia is getting worse. She has been in hospital twice in the last six months. It is likely that she is within the last year of her life. It is important to acknowledge the concerns of her family and discuss her prognosis and future goals. Her progressive cognitive and physical frailty have made her very vulnerable to minor insults. It may be difficult to prevent a pattern of recurrent hospital admissions, but there are options to de-medicalise the situation and focus more on symptom control than on longer term risk reduction. Advance care planning, involving Angela's daughter, could be used to focus on her best interests. In the event of a cardiac arrest, attempting cardiopulmonary resuscitation could not provide a beneficial outcome for Angela [see Case 10]. Completion of a 'do not attempt resuscitation' form, with discussion with her daughter, is appropriate.

Key Points

- OH is common. For older people with multi-morbidity, deprescribing is usually the key management step.
- Deciding on continuation of anticoagulation for older people with frailty and falls is not clear-cut and requires an individualised approach with shared decision-making.
- In clinical trials, antidepressant medications have not been found to be effective for people with dementia.

Further Reading

1. Gilani A, Juraschek SP, Belanger MJ, et al. Postural hypotension. *BMJ* 2021;373:n922. https://doi.org/10.1136/bmj.n922

2. National Institute for Health and Care Excellence. *Hypertension in Adults: Diagnosis and Management.* 2019. www.nice.org.uk/guidance/ng136

3. Khan F, Rahman A, Carrier M, et al. Long term risk of symptomatic recurrent venous thromboembolism after discontinuation of anticoagulant treatment for first unprovoked venous thromboembolism event: systematic review and meta-analysis. *BMJ* 2019;366:l4363 https://doi.org/10.1136/bmj.l4363

4. 2019 ESC Guidelines for the diagnosis and management of acute pulmonary embolism developed in collaboration with the European Respiratory Society (ERS). *Eur Heart J* 2020;41:543–603 https://doi.org/10.1093/eurheartj/ehz405

5. Wang W, Lessard D, Kiefe CI, et al. Differential effect of anticoagulation according to cognitive function and frailty in older patients with atrial fibrillation. *J Am Geriatr Soc.* 2023;71:394–403. https://doi.org/10.1111/jgs.18079

6. Dudas R, Malouf R, McCleery J, et al. Antidepressants for treating depression in dementia. *Cochrane Database Syst Rev* 2018;Issue 8. Art. No.: CD003944. https://doi.org/10.1002/14651858.CD003944.pub2

Case 12

David

David is a 77-year-old man who presents with a one-week history of gradually worsening shortness of breath. He describes a cough and thick secretions in his throat that he is unable to bring up. He does not have any fever, rigors, dysuria, or urinary frequency. His bowels were last open the previous morning. Recently, he had been struggling to mobilise around his home due to breathlessness. He had been discharged a week ago following a month-long admission with decompensated heart failure and COVID infection.

Past Medical History

Right arm deep vein thrombosis four years ago—commenced on apixaban
Laryngeal cancer—treated with laser resection and neck dissection four years ago
Type 2 diabetes (T2DM)
Asthma
Heart failure with preserved ejection fraction (HFpEF; 55–60% on last echocardiogram)
Upper gastrointestinal bleed—duodenal ulcer found at endoscopy six years ago
Chronic kidney disease
Non-alcoholic fatty liver disease
Hypertension

Medication

Alfacalcidol 500 ng od	Amlodipine 5 mg od
Apixaban 5 mg bd	Aspirin 75 mg od
Biphasic isophane insulin 14U AM, 12U PM	Budesonide with formoterol (160 mcg/4.5 mcg) DPI bd
Duloxetine 60 mg bd	Montelukast 10 mg n
Furosemide 40 mg od	Salbutamol inhaler as required
Omeprazole 20 mg bd	
Senna 15 mg n	

Social History

David lives alone with a carer visiting twice weekly to assist with laundry, cleaning, and shopping for microwave meals that he can heat up. He walks with a single stick in his own property but uses an electric wheelchair if he goes out. He lives in a ground floor flat without any stairs. Recently, he has been sleeping in a chair in his front room because he finds this more comfortable for his breathing. He has never smoked and doesn't drink alcohol.

Examination

Multiple scabs/scars on toes and feet. Bilateral pitting oedema and skin erythema up to the knees bilaterally. Jugular venous pulse not visible—partly due to neck scarring from laryngeal cancer treatment. Heart sounds normal, pulse irregular. Chest: globally poor inspiration, audible upper airway secretions, bi-basal chest crackles, and expiratory wheeze.

Six-Item Screener 6/6

BP 141/71 mmHg, pulse 83 bpm, oxygen saturation 93% on air, temperature 36.3°C, glucose 16.9 mmol/L, weight 124.7 kg

Investigations

Biochemistry	Value	Reference range	Haematology	Value	Reference range
Sodium	139	133–146 mmol/L	Haemoglobin	87	130–180 g/L
Potassium	4.2	3.5–5.3 mmol/L	MCV	85	82–100 fL
Urea	15.1	2.5–7.8 mmol/L	White cell count	13.2	4–11 10^9/L
Creatinine	237	64–104 umol/L	Neutrophils	10.7	2–7.5 10^9/L
C-reactive protein	134	< 5 mg/L	Platelets	222	140–400 10^9/L

Blood tests a month ago: haemoglobin 90, urea 16.3, creatinine 228, Hb_{A1C} 75; vitamin B_{12}, folate, and ferritin all in normal range
ECG—sinus rhythm 87 bpm, with atrial ectopic beats and left ventricular hypertrophy
CXR—no significant acute lesion was seen

Progress

The initial diagnosis was pneumonia with decompensation of his heart failure with preserved ejection fraction. He was treated with intravenous antibiotics and intravenous diuretics, which were both switched to oral treatments within a couple of days as his symptoms, observations, and blood tests began to improve.

David fell during his hospital stay while walking to the toilet. He bumped his head, and because he was prescribed apixaban, a CT brain scan was performed (see Figure 12.1). This showed an acute sub-dural haematoma (SDH) around the left edge of his brain. He did not have any neurological deficit. His treatment options were discussed with the local neurosurgical team, who did not think that immediate operative intervention was indicated. They recommended reversal of his anticoagulation and 48 hours of neurological observation with a view to repeat brain scanning if his condition deteriorated. If there was no change in condition, a repeat brain CT after ten days was advised.

He was treated with prothrombin complex concentrate, and his apixaban and aspirin were withheld. He also had ongoing antibiotics for his pneumonia and fluid balance optimisation.

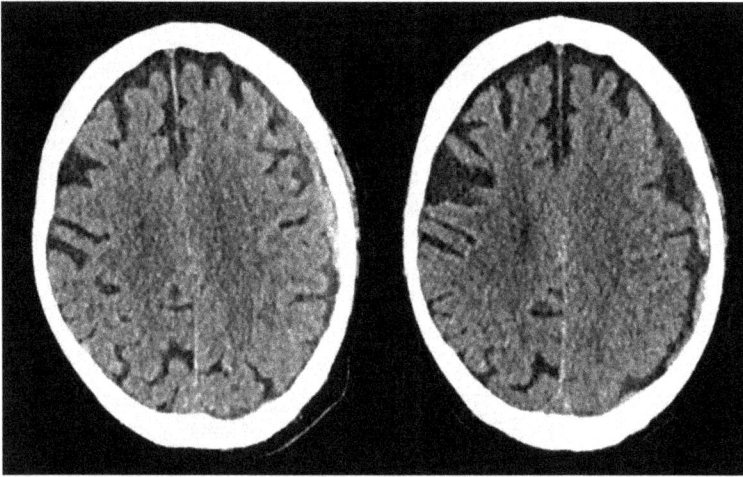

Figure 12.1 Brain CT images at first presentation and the repeat scan ten days later.

His neurological observations remained stable, but he did not return to his usual level of mobility. Repeat CT scanning at ten days showed only a minor change in the size of his SDH, and no neurosurgical intervention was deemed appropriate.

> **What interventions can reduce the risk of falling in the hospital setting?**
> **What considerations might there be about operative intervention for his SDH?**
> **Should anticoagulant treatment be restarted after traumatic SDH?**

In-patient Falls

Older people in hospital are at increased risk of falling. Higher risk is associated with cognitive impairment, previous falls, gait and balance impairment, urinary or faecal incontinence or urgency, and the use of certain medications [see Case 4]. No falls risk stratification tool has been shown to be effective at delineating risk levels in clinical trials, but when risk factors are identified, developing a personalised care plan to mitigate them is advised.[1]

Environmental approaches have a role. Guidance typically recommends ensuring appropriate lighting, flooring type, clear signage, access to a call bell, and suitable footwear. Ward cultures and practices around getting people up and moving to minimise deconditioning also help. Collaborative working between medical, nursing, and therapy staff around assessment and intervention relating to mobility (i.e. CGA) is valuable. From a specific medical perspective, on top of accurate diagnosis and treatment of acute illness, identifying whether someone is delirious or has fallen, and reviewing their medications list with a view to reducing or stopping medications that increase the risk of delirium/falling, is important. Removal of restraints (e.g. urinary catheters, intravenous drips, oxygen tubing) at the earliest opportunity allows increased independence and reduces risk of tripping. The Hospital Elder Life Program is an institutional, environmental, and clinical approach to caring for older people with frailty in hospital.[2] By undertaking CGA and developing personalised management plans, the incidence of in-patient delirium and falls was reduced.

Surgery for SDH

Emergency surgery for acute SDH with significant mass effect and cerebral oedema is a very large undertaking typically requiring craniotomy, often hemi-craniectomy and clot evacuation, followed by a time on a critical care unit and then a period of recovery and rehabilitation. It is difficult to survive and return to functional independence following this, particularly for those who were frail prior to the injury or who had a low Glasgow Coma Scale score at diagnosis. Chronic SDH surgery by contrast is simpler. It can usually be undertaken with burr-hole and drain insertion techniques, possibly under local anaesthetic. It is aimed at removal of the organised clot to alleviate persistent neurological symptoms. Predictors of poor outcome following surgery for chronic SDH include increasing age, poor functional status prior to insult, and altered consciousness prior to surgery.

Surgical outcomes tend to be best for those who are younger, fitter, and have least disability from the insult, which is the same group who have better outcomes without surgery. Without a clinical trial, we don't know for sure if or when surgery is better than a non-operative approach. Consequently, it is easy to see why very few frail older people are offered emergency surgery for acute SDH, and attempts are made to manage the situation conservatively in the initial phase. This is the reasoning behind delayed scanning, as it allows an understanding of the change in clinical and radiological picture over time to determine whether operative intervention might be feasible and of value. It can be confusing for patients, relatives, and staff, however, if we are repeating a scan to see if things have changed inside the skull regardless of how the person is recovering. And especially confusing if no one thinks brain surgery would be wise. It is usually better to determine the potential value of undertaking any test using all available information alongside the goals of the person themself.

Should Anticoagulant Treatment be Restarted after Traumatic SDH?

A major haemorrhage of any kind should lead to a careful assessment of risk and benefit of all medications that alter the likelihood of bleeding. In Case 11, we reviewed the risk and benefit of anticoagulation for venous thrombo-embolism. Regarding traumatic intracerebral haemorrhage, there is the particular concern of risk of falls. With recent national guidelines in the UK advocating for urgent CT scanning in those people on anticoagulants who bang their heads, the therapeutic burden of anticoagulation should include recurrent emergency department attendances for scans which many find to be exhausting and distressing. In David's case, a fall led to the SDH and so the risk of falling factors into the risk-benefit analysis. If it is possible to significantly reduce his risk of falling (e.g. deprescribing medications, improving gait and balance, or reducing environmental hazards), then it could favour restarting apixaban after recovery. If the risk of falling remains high, there would be a stronger argument for stopping the anticoagulant altogether.

What about David?

Reviewing David's records, it was discovered that the co-prescription of aspirin and apixaban was a prescribing error. The apixaban was initiated for deep vein thrombosis, but he was already taking aspirin for primary vascular prevention. This should have been stopped, as the combination was not indicated and poses higher risk of bleeding adverse events. David was also co-prescribed amlodipine and furosemide. This is a well-recognised prescribing cascade. If amlodipine is causing leg oedema, then an alternative BP-lowering medication may be more suitable. Given his recent fall, it is important to measure his BP both lying and standing. If he has a postural drop, then the lower value obtained should be used to guide antihypertensive medication prescribing. His Hb_{A1C} is raised at 75, but this may not be a reliable indicator of his glucose control due to having anaemia. Monitoring his blood glucose is more likely to be a useful guide for his insulin dose. His anaemia is likely to be caused by renal impairment. Given his combination of T2DM and HFpEF, he may be suitable for treatment with an SGLT2 inhibitor.

The potential risk and benefit of reintroducing anticoagulation for David will be affected by how he recovers in terms of independence following these latest insults. Prior to admission, his mobility was limited, but he had managed to retain his independence. If his cognition remains poor and his mobility does not recover, then his life expectancy will be impacted. Overall, this would reduce the potential benefit and increase the potential risk of the medication. Shared decision-making conversations of this level of complexity are best undertaken as a relationship develops over time between the person, their carer, and the clinical team.

David has mild frailty (CFS 5). Recent difficulty with breathing has led to him sleeping in a chair. Treating his chest infection and adjusting the management of his heart failure may improve the situation. If he were able to optimise his weight, then this could also help. The physiotherapy team can assess to ensure he has the most suitable mobility aid. As he has not returned to his previous level of mobility so far, a period of rehabilitation is appropriate. The occupational therapy team can ensure he has the right adaptations and equipment to support him when he does return home.

Key Points

- Older people in hospital are at risk of falling.
- Personalised approaches around medications, institutional approaches around environmental layout, and cultural practices around deconditioning avoidance can be employed to reduce risk.
- Emergency surgery for subdural haematoma evacuation is rarely indicated for older people with frailty, and early conversations about realistic outcomes can be helpful.

Further Reading

1. National Institute for Health and Care Excellence. *Falls: Assessment and Prevention of Falls in Older People.* 2013. www.nice.org.uk/guidance/cg161
2. Hshieh TT, Yang T, Gartaganis SL et al. Hospital elder life program: systematic review and meta-analysis of effectiveness. *Am J Geriatr Psychiatry* 2018;26:1015–33. https://doi.org/10.1016/j.jagp.2018.06.007

Case 13

Veronica

Veronica is an 86-year-old former civil servant. She was referred to clinic having fallen several times over the last six months. Two of these occurred when she was sitting on a chair, and she feels that she simply lost balance and fell forwards onto the floor. She had another fall in the kitchen, and she was unclear why. She sometimes gets light-headedness if she stands up quickly. She has urinary incontinence and urgency episodes and gets up at each night to pass urine two or three times. On several occasions, falls have occurred when going to the toilet overnight. She does not feel that the trospium or mirabegron she has been prescribed has helped her symptoms, and she has already reduced the trospium to once a day, which has not made any difference. In the last three months, she has also had occasional episodes of faecal incontinence. She has been wearing continence pads that she has purchased herself. She finds this very embarrassing to discuss. She passes a bowel motion once or twice each day, which has not changed recently. She describes her motions as having a normal consistency. Over the last year, she has also noticed swelling of both of her ankles.

Past Medical History

Hypertension
Ischaemic heart disease
Overactive bladder

Medication

Amlodipine 5 mg od	Aspirin 75 mg od
Atenolol 25 mg od	Bendroflumethiazide 2.5 mg od
Mirabegron MR 50 mg od	Omeprazole 20 mg od
Simvastatin 20 mg at night	Trospium 20 mg bd (currently taking od)

Social History

Veronica lives alone in a downstairs flat. She tends to furniture walk around her property and mobilises outdoors with a stick. She has not been outside alone for over a year. She is independent with all her personal care. She orders shopping online, and her neighbours help with any extra items she might need.

DOI: 10.1201/9781003582007-13

Examination

She has bilateral pitting leg oedema below the knees. Her JVP was not elevated. She has a soft systolic heart murmur. Her chest was clear. Abdomen soft and non-tender.

Six-Item Screener 4/6

BP 134/70 mmHg while lying and 144/77 mmHg one minute after standing, pulse 67 bpm, oxygen saturation 95% on air, temperature 36.6°C

Investigations

Biochemistry	Value	Reference range	Haematology	Value	Reference range
Sodium	136	133–146 mmol/L	Haemoglobin	126	115–165 g/L
Potassium	3.6	3.5–5.3 mmol/L	MCV	85	82–100 fL
Urea	6.1	2.5–7.8 mmol/L	White cell count	6.8	4–11 10^9/L
Creatinine	77	49–90 umol/L	Platelets	303	140–400 10^9/L
C-reactive protein	2	< 5 mg/L			

Liver blood tests, calcium, and glucose all normal

Why is Veronica falling over?
What is the cause of her urinary symptoms, and what can be done?
What is the cause of her faecal incontinence, and what can be done?

Veronica's Falls

Veronica's falls do not all sound the same. On some occasions, she seems to lose balance while sitting in a chair. On other occasions, she feels light-headed on standing. It is likely that several underlying mechanisms co-exist. These are likely to include gait and balance impairment and orthostatic hypotension (OH). This latter problem is not excluded by a single lying/standing blood pressure measurement not showing a drop. Urinary urgency may make her rush to get to the toilet, increasing her risk of falling on the way. The added weight of leg oedema may also affect her mobility. There is some evidence of cognitive impairment too. Adverse effects of medications may contribute to several of these problems.

Urinary Incontinence

Incontinence in older people with frailty is likely to be multifactorial. Continence requires brain and body to function well enough to get to the toilet reliably every time. Cognitive impairment can lead to loss of awareness of the need to go, difficulty finding the toilet (especially in unfamiliar environments), and sometimes socially inappropriate behaviour. Physical function impairment can affect accessing the toilet in a timely way, including removing enough clothing. In younger and less frail people, the focus of continence assessments is based around bladder and pelvic floor function and characteristics of the urine. In geriatric medicine, the cause of incontinence requires a less 'cystoscopic' approach; problems relate to the whole body and surrounding environment, often more than the bladder. Interventions addressing polypharmacy, mobility, cognition, and bowel health can have significant impact in the management of urinary continence.

Urinary incontinence can be classified into the following subtypes (but more than one may co-exist):

- Urge—strong bladder contractions making the person rush to the toilet or leak large volumes of urine
- Stress—pelvic floor weakness leading to leakage of small volumes of urine on coughing, straining, or positional change
- Overflow—continually leaking small volumes of urine due to either bladder outflow obstruction (e.g. constipation or a large prostate) or neurological weakness of the bladder (e.g. diabetic neuropathy)
- Functional—difficulty accessing toileting facilities due to physical, cognitive, or environmental issues

Some physical conditions can increase urine output—e.g. hyperglycaemia and hypercalcaemia—and heart failure can lead to nocturia (i.e. reabsorption of peripheral oedema when lying flat in bed). Some medications can be unhelpful, for example:

- Anticholinergics—overflow (i.e. constipation and bladder relaxation)
- Alpha blockers—stress (pelvic floor muscle relaxation)
- Psychotropics—reduced ability/awareness to access toilet
- Constipating drugs—leading to faecal impaction
- Cholinesterase inhibitors—urge (i.e. pro-cholinergic action)
- Drugs causing peripheral oedema (e.g. calcium channel blockers, dopamine agonists, gabapentinoids)
- Diuretics—especially loop diuretics, need to rush to toilet in the hours after a dose

Anticholinergic drugs (e.g. oxybutynin, tolterodine, and solifenacin) can be used for urge incontinence but are associated with a high risk of adverse effects in older people with frailty—especially cognitive impairment, constipation, and falls. Their effect size for reducing incontinence episodes is only small.[1] If your patient is already taking one, then ask them if they find it beneficial and if they still need to wear containment pads.

The usual initial management steps for urinary incontinence affecting older people with frailty are listed next:

- Look for any underlying cause(s)—i.e. perform CGA.
- Consider a bladder scan to exclude overflow.
- Avoid catheters—plan for removal if inserted during current admission.
- Do not start an anticholinergic medication.

For Veronica, her incontinence is likely to be predominantly due to her declining mobility. Perhaps predictably, medications to relax the bladder have not had a significant symptomatic benefit and may simply risk adverse effects. Trospium has strong anticholinergic effects and could impair cognitive function [see Case 9] as well as potentially causing a dry mouth and constipation. Mirabegron is a beta 3 agonist and could increase blood pressure and heart rate and has little clinical trial evidence to suggest usefulness for older people with frailty. Both should be considered for deprescribing if not improving her symptoms. Veronica has already started reducing trospium.

Nocturia

Older people are more prone to nocturia. The physiological process that reduces the quantity of urine that we produce overnight becomes less effective (i.e. diurnal variation in vasopressin secretion). Also, our bladders become less elastic and are less good at storing urine. It is common for older people to get up to pass urine once or twice overnight. This may also be partly because our sleep becomes more broken due to old age, and some people go to the toilet when they wake up 'just in case'.

We can reduce the amount of urine we produce overnight by having our last non-alcoholic drink at least three hours before bedtime and avoiding everything with a diuretic effect, such as alcohol or caffeinated drinks. The advice is not to reduce total fluid intake, and risk dehydration, but instead drink the appropriate volume of fluid earlier in their day. The amount of salt in our diet also seems to affect nocturia, with lower salt intakes reducing symptoms.[2] Salt reduction may also improve the control of hypertension. Salt can be added to foods but is also present in high quantities in many processed or packeted foods and dispersible medication formulations.

Peripheral oedema accumulates during the day because of gravity. Lying down in bed overnight usually improves the oedema because a volume of the fluid is reabsorbed and converted into urine. Reducing oedema can reduce nocturnal urine production. There are a variety of potential causes of oedema [see Case 4], and the best treatment for each person depends on the likely cause. In Veronica's case, her peripheral oedema is likely to be partly due to amlodipine. Deprescribing this medication is likely to be helpful. An alternative agent to control her blood pressure or angina may need to be considered.

Improving access to the toilet overnight may also help. A bedside commode should be considered. For some, handheld urinals at the bedside might be enough. For people with restricted mobility, wearing a continence pad overnight can avoid the necessity to get up overnight but isn't acceptable to everyone. Often as a last resort, urinary catheters are sometimes tried for very troublesome nocturia but have their own potential problems [see Case 18].

Faecal Incontinence

Faecal incontinence in older people with frailty is often associated with cognitive impairment and a reduced awareness of the need to go to the toilet. Sometimes it can be induced by diarrhoea or constipation, which can lead to faecal impaction and overflow diarrhoea. Impaired mobility may also contribute. So, a combination of things can precipitate faecal incontinence. Obtaining a history, with the help of collateral when appropriate, gives clues to the underlying reason. For example, some people lose awareness of the need to go, pelvic floor weakness can lead to incontinence on postural change, and cognitive impairment or mood disorders are relevant for others. There may be associated diarrhoea or constipation. Stool charts and physical examination can help this aspect of assessment.

For people with diarrhoea, exclude bowel infections and check for any medications that could be causative. Assuming overflow diarrhoea is not suspected, laxatives should be withheld. Several medication types can also cause diarrhoea, possibly via microscopic colitis. These include proton pump inhibitors and selective serotonin reuptake inhibitors. Once these have all been considered, a trial of a constipating medication, such as loperamide, may be appropriate. Constipation is discussed in Case 18. When associated, any faecal impaction should be cleared, which may require enemas. Improving mobility and toilet access should be attempted. For people with cognitive impairment, a regular toileting regime may help (i.e. proactively helping the person to the toilet at selected times of the day).

What about Veronica?

Some of Veronica's symptoms are suggestive of an element of OH. Her peripheral oedema is almost certainly related to her amlodipine. For both reasons, after discussion of the risks and benefits, amlodipine was discontinued. This medication was taken for BP control. She had not experienced any angina in the last few years. The medications she takes for urinary incontinence do not seem to be having any positive effect and could expose her to adverse effects. She agreed with a trial of discontinuation.

After she had stopped taking amlodipine, a 24-hour BP monitor was arranged to get more information about her BP control. Given the suspected OH, decisions about her future BP management should also include measurements taken one minute after standing [see Case 11]. Physiotherapy assessment led to provision of a new two-wheeled walking frame. The physiotherapy team also arranged follow-up with some gait and balance group work exercise sessions. An occupational therapist visited her at home to look for environmental risk factors for falling.

Coming off amlodipine should help to reduce her leg oedema. This may help her mobility and reduce nocturia. Veronica did not drink any alcohol but had got into the habit of having a cup of tea before going to bed. She was educated on why this would not help either her sleeping, due to caffeine content, or her need to pass urine overnight. She was advised to avoid drinking any fluid in the three hours before bedtime. Ways that she might reduce salt in her diet were discussed. The occupational therapy team also provided her with a bedside commode to make toilet access easier for her overnight.

Key Points

- Any medication taken for symptomatic benefit that doesn't reduce symptoms should be reviewed and considered for deprescribing/change.
- Impaired mobility, falls, and incontinence often co-exist.
- The causes of incontinence often lie outside of the bladder or bowel and may be multifactorial. CGA is the correct approach for older people with frailty.

Further Reading

1. Stoniute A, Madhuvrata P, Still M, et al. Oral anticholinergic drugs versus placebo or no treatment for managing overactive bladder syndrome in adults. *Cochrane Database Syst Rev* 2023;Issue 5. Art. No.: CD003781. https://doi.org/10.1002/14651858.CD003781.pub3
2. Monaghan TF, Michelson KP, Wu ZD, et al. Sodium restriction improves nocturia in patients at a cardiology clinic. *J Clin Hypertens* 2020;22:633–8. https://doi.org/10.1111/jch.13829

Case 14

Mohammed

Mohammed is an 83-year-old retired dentist who came to hospital after two falls. He was testing out his new mobility scooter when he hit a low kerb and fell out onto his right-hand side. He was able to get himself up off the floor and get back to his home. Once inside, he had another fall in the bathroom, again onto his right side. Since then, he has been unable to mobilise due to a right hip pain. He does not report any other injuries and is clear that he didn't bump his head with either fall.

Past Medical History

Parkinsonism—unclear aetiology
CT brain scan showed global atrophy and small vessel disease with some old lacunar infarcts.

> DAT scan suggested possible dementia with Lewy bodies.
> Known to falls and Parkinson's disease services (initially labelled as essential tremor/ vascular parkinsonism). Treatment trial with levodopa started two years ago, no improvement noted in relevant clinic letters.

Vascular dementia (MOCA 16/30 one year ago)
Previous bilateral hip surgery—total hip replacements for osteoarthritis
Orthostatic hypotension (OH)—investigations under falls team
Central retinal artery occlusion nine years ago
COPD
Depression

> Has been taking two antidepressants for > 6 years. Seven years ago, he underwent an in-patient psychiatry assessment shortly after the death of his wife (low mood, suicidal thoughts, reduced oral intake). He doesn't have current psychiatry follow-up.

Ischaemic heart disease

Medication

Atorvastatin 40 mg tablets od	Bisoprolol 2.5 mg od
Budesonide 320 mcg/formoterol 9 mcg DPI bd	Clopidogrel 75 mg tablets od
Co-careldopa 125 mg at 8 AM, 12 noon and 4 PM	Co-beneldopa 12.5 mg/50 mg dispersible as required

DOI: 10.1201/9781003582007-14

Glyceryl trinitrate 400 mcg sublingual spray as required	Hydroxocobalamin 1 mg/1 ml injection three-monthly
Melatonin 2 mg MR n	Mirtazapine 30 mg at night
Salbutamol 200 mcg DPI as required	Sertraline 150 mg od

Social History

Mohammed lives alone in a sheltered accommodation, which consists of a first-floor flat with lift access and 24-hour warden support. Carers come in twice a day to help with getting washed and dressed/undressed. He sometimes uses a two-wheeled walking frame around his property but at times supports himself by holding on to the furniture instead. He quit smoking nine years ago and has never drunk alcohol. He has two sons, who both live locally, but they tend to be very busy with work and their own families.

Examination

He is alert. No focal neurological deficit and normal tone in limbs. Heart sounds normal, no oedema, and chest is clear. Abdomen soft and non-tender. Reasonable range of movement in both hips but some pain and bruising over his right hip.

Six-Item Screener 1/6

4AT 3/12

BP 158/75 mmHg, pulse 58 bpm, oxygen saturation 95% on air, temperature 36.4°C

Investigations

Biochemistry	Value	Reference range	Haematology	Value	Reference range
Sodium	139	133–146 mmol/L	Haemoglobin	97	130–180 g/L
Potassium	4.6	3.5–5.3 mmol/L	MCV	71	82–100 fL
Urea	11.1	2.5–7.8 mmol/L	White cell count	12.8	4–11 10⁹/L
Creatinine	100	64–104 umol/L	Neutrophils	9.8	2–7.5 10⁹/L
C-reactive protein	9	< 5 mg/L	Platelets	198	140–400 10⁹/L

Liver blood tests and calcium normal

Six months ago: urea 10.5, creatinine 94, haemoglobin 115, MCV 82, vitamin B_{12} 145 (150–1000 ng/L; commenced on hydroxocobalamin injections afterwards), folate 3.9 (2–18.8) ug/L, ferritin 19 (12–250) ug/L

ECG—sinus rhythm, 50 bpm, no acute changes

Pelvic X-ray—previous bilateral hip replacements, no fracture

How do we distinguish different causes of parkinsonism?

What about his microcytic anaemia?

Would you consider changing any of his medications?

What are the considerations for discharge planning?

Parkinsonism

Parkinsonism is a term for having some clinical features of Parkinson's disease (PD). It can be caused by a variety of pathologies and is typically defined as having two or more of the following: bradykinesia, gait disturbance, rigidity, and/or tremor. PD results from loss of dopaminergic neurons in the basal ganglia. The classic tremor of PD is most obvious at rest with the thumb moving across the palm in a 'pill-rolling' manner. Parkinsonism due to other pathologies is much more common than PD in older people with frailty, who are also likely to have multiple pathologies within their brains, making accurate diagnosis more challenging. Even when PD pathology is present, co-existence of other pathologies could reduce the benefit and/or increase the risk of harm from treatments for PD. Brain lesions causing parkinsonism include cerebrovascular disease, other neurodegenerative conditions (e.g. Alzheimer's dementia), and drug-induced (e.g. history of antipsychotic drug exposure). Non-PD neurodegenerative movement disorders are possible but less common (e.g. dementia with Lewy bodies [DLB], multiple system atrophy [MSA], or progressive supranuclear palsy [PSP]). Clinical features that can help to distinguish between PD and other causes of parkinsonism are outlined in Table 14.1. Sometimes the diagnosis becomes clearer as the condition progresses, and follow-up in a specialist movement disorders clinic increases the accuracy of diagnosis over time.

A dopamine active transporter (DAT) scan uses [1,2,3]I-FP-CIT single-photon emission computed tomography (SPECT) to assist the diagnosis of parkinsonism. Reduced uptake in the basal ganglia should be found in people with PD, DLB, MSA, or PSP. Reduced uptake should not be found with drug-induced parkinsonism or essential tremor, so its primary

Table 14.1 Clinical Features that Can Help to Distinguish Between PD and Parkinsonism of Different Cause

	Parkinson's disease	Non-PD parkinsonism
Onset	Unilateral Presentation uncommon after age 80	Bilateral and symmetrical Common after age 80
Progression	Slowly progressive	Often more rapid, sometimes 'stepwise' decline
'Pill-rolling' tremor	Common	Rare
Gait	Stooped forward, narrow based, loss of arm swing, festinating	More upright, broad-based, small stepping [see Case 20]
Other features	Good response to levodopa therapy Motor features most obvious in arms	Minimal response to levodopa Early cognitive impairment and/or falls Axial rigidity or motor features most obvious in legs

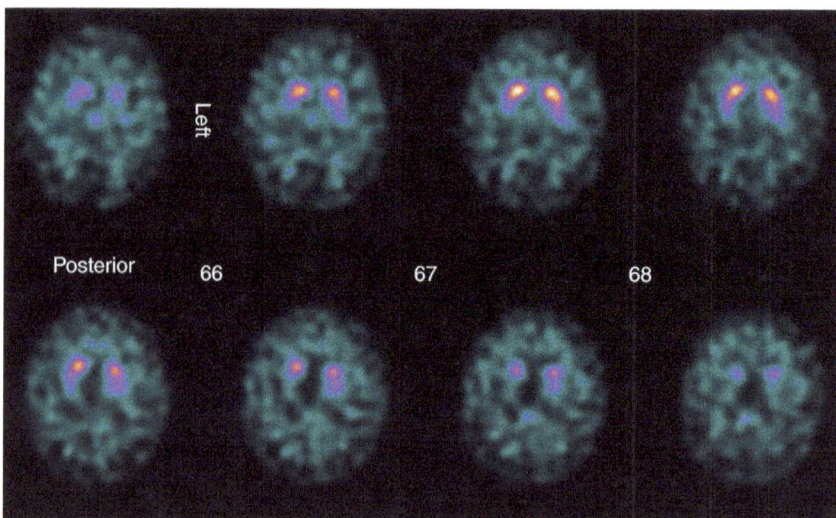

Figure 14.1 DAT scan images showing some asymmetry of uptake in the basal ganglia.

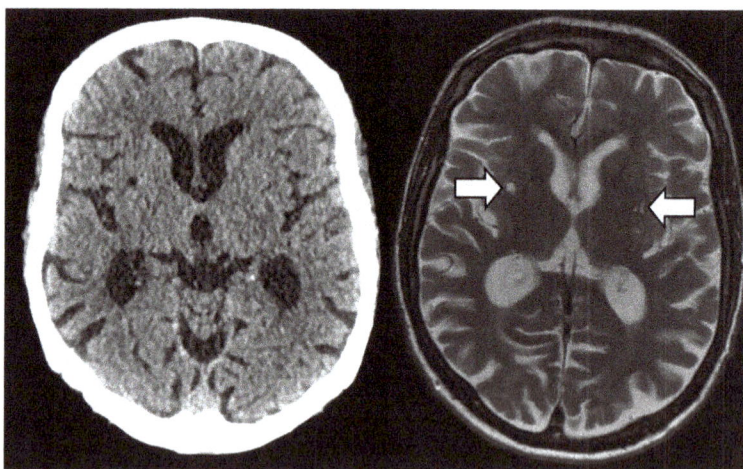

Figure 14.2 CT and MRI brain scans showing vascular lesions in the basal ganglia (arrows).

role is to rule out PD, DLB, MSA, or PSP in people with parkinsonism thought to be drug-induced or essential tremor. The technique is less precise at distinguishing PD/DLB/MSA/PSP from vascular parkinsonism or Alzheimer's dementia. Its role in diagnosis for older people with multi-morbidity is much less clear, largely because cerebral atrophy and small vessel disease become ubiquitous. Mohammed's DAT scan (see Figure 14.1) shows reduced uptake bilaterally at the putamen but more marked on the right than left. These areas appear to correspond with old lacunar infarcts and underlying small vessel disease on his CT and MRI brain scans (see Figure 14.2), suggesting that cerebrovascular disease could explain the DAT scan appearance.

For all forms of parkinsonism except PD, dopaminergic medications have little, if any, benefit. Potential harms include cognitive impairment, constipation, and OH. There are no disease-modifying drugs for PD. Levodopa, the active component of co-careldopa, provides the greatest symptomatic relief of the available medicines. If no symptomatic benefit has been found, despite a reasonable dose, then a slow, gradual withdrawal, with monitoring to ensure no deterioration in motor symptoms, could be tried. For Mohammed, his parkinsonism seems most likely to be predominantly vascular in aetiology. There has been no clear symptomatic benefit, and he is at high risk of confusion and falls. A trial of slowly reducing his co-careldopa dose with careful monitoring would be reasonable. This should be discussed with him, his sons, and the PD service who already know him.

Normal Pressure Hydrocephalus

Sometimes normal pressure hydrocephalus is suggested as a cause of the 'classical triad' of cognitive impairment, gait impairment, and urinary incontinence. The validity of this diagnostic term has been questioned.[1] In the absence of an obstructed cerebrospinal fluid system, there is no reason for cerebral ventricles to become enlarged. It probably usually represents a misdiagnosis of cerebral atrophy due to combined neurodegenerative and vascular lesions in older people. The authors suggest avoidance of this label.

Microcytic Anaemia

Mohammed has developed microcytic anaemia within the last year. The recent development excludes longstanding conditions, such as thalassaemia. Iron-deficiency anaemia (IDA) is almost certainly the cause, which can be confirmed by checking serum ferritin concentration. Although serum ferritin can be affected by inflammation. Serum ferritin < 30 suggests IDA and > 150 makes it unlikely, even in the presence of an inflammatory condition.[2] Results in the range 30 to 150, in the presence of inflammation, represent a grey area. If in doubt, then a trial of iron replacement with monitoring of response is an option. In the absence of an alternative explanation for IDA, e.g. frank haematuria, slow gastrointestinal (GI) blood loss is the most likely cause in men and post-menopausal women. Some people have more than one contributing lesion.

Upper and lower GI endoscopy is the usual way to look for underlying problems. In a series of people having endoscopies for IDA, a relevant lesion was detected in 36% of the sub-group aged 80 and over.[3] In 15%, cancer was detected (over 80% of these found in the lower GI tract), 11% had an inflammatory cause (e.g. peptic ulcer disease, oesophagitis, diverticulitis), 5% had angiodysplasia, 4% had a benign tumour (e.g. a bowel polyp), and 1% were diagnosed with coeliac disease. Serology for coeliac disease is less reliable in older people and duodenal biopsy may be better.[2] Faecal immunochemical testing (FIT) is sometimes used to help risk stratify suspected colorectal cancer, but the sensitivity may only be around 83%, meaning cases could be missed.[2]

GI endoscopies are invasive tests and not well tolerated in some older people with frailty. CT colonography, which requires bowel prep and inflation of the colon with carbon dioxide, is less invasive and sedation not required. This technique can help diagnose some structural lesions (i.e. not angiodysplasia) but can't offer any therapy (e.g. polyp removal) or biopsy.

Contrast CT, without bowel prep, can visualise some large lesions, but is that of real value? A person who is not fit enough for an endoscopy is probably not fit enough for any kind of surgical procedure.

For Mohammed, his physical and cognitive frailty make it likely that endoscopic tests would be burdensome. An assessment of his attitude towards these tests and his capacity to consent is appropriate. Data previously discussed suggest there is a 64% chance that endoscopies wouldn't detect the source of his anaemia. If a structural lesion was detected, then would it lead to further intervention? One option would be to take a more pragmatic approach without further testing. Mohammed has been taking clopidogrel for IHD and a central retinal artery embolism that occurred nine years ago. Around 64 people with IHD need to be treated with an antiplatelet drug per year to prevent one adverse vascular event.[4] Taking clopidogrel has no effect on the progression of vascular dementia. Clopidogrel will increase his risk of bleeding, both from the GI tract and a small increased risk of intracranial bleeding with falls. Now that he has microcytic anaemia, the risk-benefit ratio of clopidogrel has altered. He is also prescribed a serotonin-specific reuptake inhibitor, sertraline, which is associated with an increased risk of GI bleeding.

A range of options exist. One possibility is to do nothing. He is unlikely to be symptomatic with mild anaemia, and this was not the cause of his admission. But things will probably continue to get worse. He could have upper and lower GI endoscopies to try to identify and treat the source. Alternatively, one or more of stopping clopidogrel, reducing the dose of sertraline (possibly aiming to slowly wean off), starting a proton-pump inhibitor (in case of peptic ulcer disease), and iron replacement could help. Regarding iron replacement, the oral route is usually tried first. Low-dose supplementation (e.g. ferrous sulfate 200 mg on alternate days) is as effective as higher-dose supplementation with fewer adverse effects (e.g. constipation). If not tolerated, intravenous iron supplementation is an option.

Medication Changes

We have already discussed Mohammed's use of co-careldopa and clopidogrel. He is also prescribed two different antidepressants. This type of medication has not been found to be beneficial for people with dementia who appear low in mood [see Case 11], but Mohammed has a history of depression that predates his dementia diagnosis. He has been on these medications for over six years. We talked about sertraline and GI bleeding risk. Mirtazapine has some anticholinergic effects and could worsen his cognition. Both antidepressants could precipitate OH. If mood symptoms are not a current key concern, then a gradual dose reduction could be considered. Input from the psychiatry team could help. Melatonin is only recommended for short-term use, up to 13 weeks. How effective has it been for his symptoms? The use of statin medications is discussed in Case 19. Taking fewer tablets may reduce his risk of future falls. Measuring lying and standing blood pressures could help with therapeutic decisions.

People with cognitive impairment can struggle with inhaler use, and their technique should be checked. Dry powder inhalers don't require coordination of actuation with breathing in but do require a forceful inhalation to get the medication deep into the lungs [see Case 22]. Mohammed might do better with a multi-dose inhaler and a spacer. The steroid component, budesonide, in his inhaler could increase his risk of developing pneumonia. If he hasn't had frequent COPD exacerbations, then switching to an inhaler with a long-acting beta agonist alone, or in combination with a long-acting muscarinic antagonist, could be tried.

Discharge Planning

Mohammed is moderately frail (CFS 6). As he lives alone and has cognitive impairment, medication adherence could be an issue. His carers could assist him with medication-taking. The care package may need to be adjusted depending on how frequently drugs are taken. A multi-dose administration aid can assist this process but is not suitable for all medications, e.g. inhalers.

Although no fracture was detected, pain is limiting Mohammed's mobility. He is likely to need analgesia and physiotherapy input to regain usual function. A period of rehabilitation, either in a dedicated unit or within his own home, may be required. If he is commenced on an opioid for pain, then he is at his risk of developing constipation, and co-prescription of a laxative is likely to be appropriate. Proactive efforts to wean off opiates as his pain improves will reduce the risk of longer-term issues relating to chronic opioid use.

Because of his physical frailty and cognitive impairment, he will continue to be at risk of future falls. A personal care alarm button, worn as a necklace or watch, could enable him to summon help, but he might forget to use it. Going into a care home would mean someone would be available if he fell over but would not stop him from falling. It's unclear whether he can safely use his mobility scooter. It was new to him when he crashed it, and perhaps his skills will improve with practice. Maybe his sons could supervise him initially and reach a consensus together. Support from voluntary organisations relating to parkinsonism or dementia could help him and his sons in dealing with the practicalities and psychological stresses of his increasing dependency on others and support him to continue to engage with his community.

Key Points

- Parkinsonism due to other pathologies is much more common than PD in older people with frailty.
- 'Normal pressure hydrocephalus' is likely to represent a misdiagnosis of cerebral atrophy due to combined neurodegenerative and vascular lesions in older people.
- GI endoscopy for iron-deficiency anaemia detects a causative lesion in around 36% of people aged over 80.

Further Reading

1. Espay AJ, Da Prat GA, Dwivedi AK, et al. Deconstructing normal pressure hydrocephalus: ventriculomegaly as early sign of neurodegeneration. *Ann Neurol* 2017;82:503–13. https://doi.org/10.1002/ana.25046

2. Snook J, Bhala N, Beales ILP, et al. British Society of Gastroenterology guidelines for the management of iron deficiency anaemia in adults. *Gut* 2021;70:2030–51. https://doi.org/10.1136/gutjnl-2021–325210

3. Stone H, Almilaji O, John C, et al. The dedicated iron deficiency anaemia clinic: a 15-year experience. *Frontline Gastroenterol* 2022;13:20–4. https://doi.org/10.1136/flgastro-2020–101470

4. Antithrombotic Trialists' Collaboration. Collaborative meta-analysis of randomised trials of antiplatelet therapy for prevention of death, myocardial infarction, and stroke in high risk patients. *BMJ* 2002;324:71–86. https://doi.org/10.1136/bmj.324.7329.71

Harold

Harold is a 90-year-old man who used to work in the shipyards. He came to hospital with his wife, Margaret, and daughter, Julie. He had not been feeling well for a few days. He describes malaise, no appetite, not drinking much, little urine output, and a cough producing yellow sputum. He had not seen any blood in the sputum. He does not usually have a cough. On the morning of admission, he couldn't catch his breath. An ambulance was called, and the paramedics found his temperature to be 38.3°C. His long-term urinary catheter had been changed four days previously but with no apparent complications. By the time he was seen in hospital, he was feeling a bit better but still had very little energy. He had managed to drink about 500 ml of water so far that day. He had not missed any of his usual medications.

Past Medical History

Pleural plaques, possible asbestosis
Prostate cancer—diagnosed five years ago, radical radiotherapy, no hormone treatment, recent biochemical recurrence (prostate-specific antigen 21 ng/ml [normal < 4.0])
Benign prostatic hyperplasia—long-term urinary catheter
Hypertension
Epilepsy
Ischaemic heart disease (IHD)
'Do not attempt resuscitation' from completed and ward-based treatment decision during previous hospital admission

Medication

Aspirin 75 mg od	Atenolol 50 mg bd
Losartan 100 mg od	Simvastatin 40 mg n
Sodium valproate MR 400 mg bd	Solifenacin 5 mg od
Tamsulosin MR 400 mcg od	

Social History

Harold lives with his wife, daughter, and grandson in a two-storey house with stairs and bilateral banister rails. He has a pendent-worn personal care alarm. He usually mobilises around the property with a two-wheeled walking frame (he has one upstairs and one downstairs). He can do the stairs independently but slowly. He does not have any formal

DOI: 10.1201/9781003582007-15

package of care. He is independent with personal care, but his daughter does most of the cooking, cleaning, laundry, and shopping.

Examination

He is alert, chatty, and talking in full sentences. Pulse is regular, and heart sounds normal. There are bi-basal crackles in his chest. Abdomen soft and non-tender. No palpable bladder. Concentrated urine in the catheter bag. His calves are soft and non-tender with mild pitting oedema.

Six-Item Screener 2/6

4AT 3/12

BP 136/65 mmHg, pulse 52 bpm, oxygen saturation 95% on air, temperature 37.0°C initially, and 38.1°C when repeated an hour later

Investigations

Biochemistry	Value	Reference range	Haematology	Value	Reference range
Sodium	137	133–146 mmol/L	Haemoglobin	132	130–180 g/L
Potassium	4.9	3.5–5.3 mmol/L	MCV	91	82–100 fL
Urea	6.8	2.5–7.8 mmol/L	White cell count	17.3	4–11 10⁹/L
Creatinine	119	64–104 umol/L	Neutrophils	14.6	2.5–7 10⁹/L
C-reactive protein	153	< 5 mg/L	Platelets	365	140–400 10⁹/L

ECG—sinus rhythm, 55 bpm

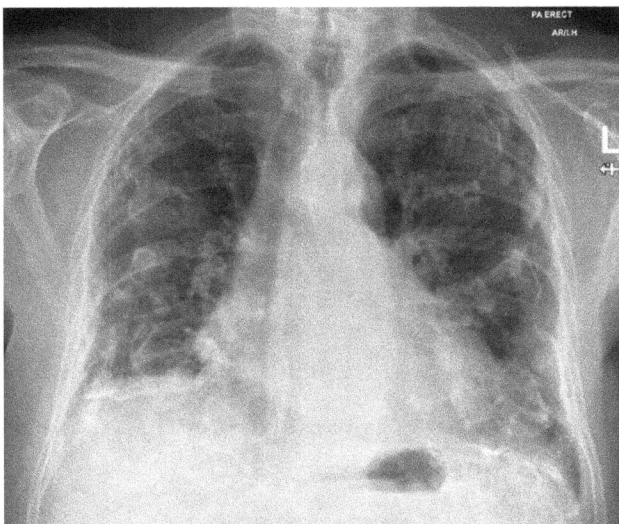

Figure 15.1 Chest X-ray showing widespread pleural plaques.

Progress

Harold was diagnosed with a chest infection and started on broad-spectrum intravenous antibiotics and intravenous fluids. Subsequent results for blood and urine cultures did not show any growth. While still in hospital two days later, Harold suddenly became very out of breath when walking back from the toilet. He was helped into his bed and positioned in an upright seated position. He grabbed hold of the bedrails and was using accessory muscles to help him breathe. Crackles were heard throughout his chest. He had been switched from intravenous to oral antibiotics earlier that day.

Observations

BP 162/85 mmHg, pulse 71 bpm, oxygen saturation 94% on 40% oxygen via a mask, temperature 35.6°C, respiratory rate 36/min

Blood Test Results from Earlier that Day

Haemoglobin 114, WCC 6.9, C-reactive protein 104

It was felt that he had developed pulmonary oedema. He was given 40 mg intravenous furosemide. An ECG and chest X-ray were repeated (see Figures 15.2 and 15.3). A serum troponin T test was sent. This showed a raised concentration of 521 ng/L (normal < 14). He was given a dose of subcutaneous fondaparinux. A repeat troponin T test three hours later had risen further to 628. A diagnosis of non-ST elevation myocardial infarction (NSTEMI) was made.

What is the optimal medical management for Harold's NSTEMI?
Would you make any changes to his other medications?

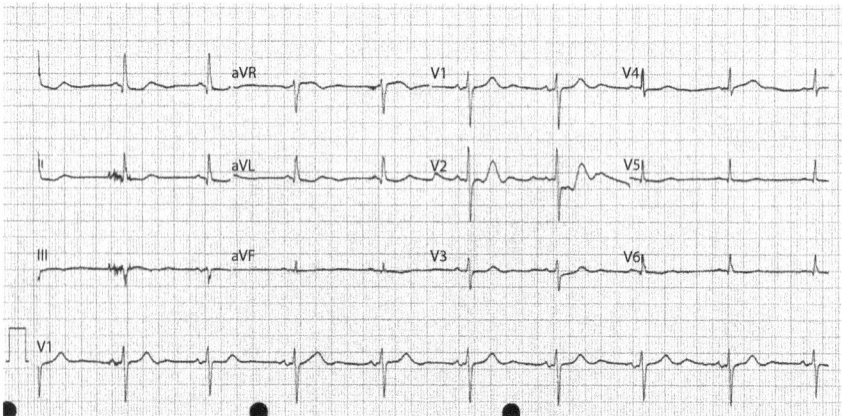

Figure 15.2 The second ECG shows that he has developed a right bundle branch block.

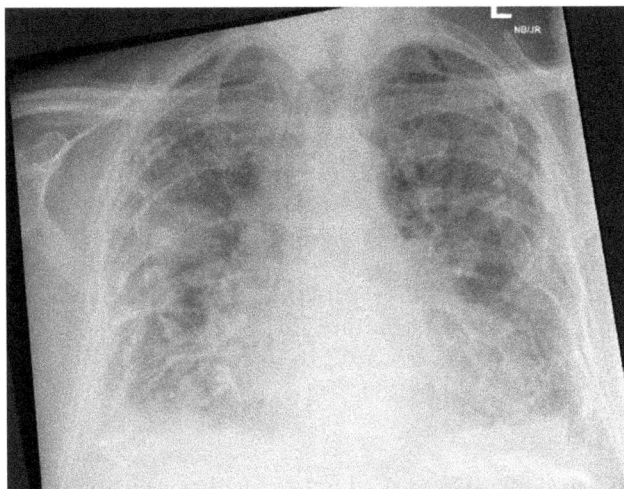

Figure 15.3 The repeat chest X-ray shows generalised increased shadowing in both lung fields, consistent with acute pulmonary oedema.

Managing Acute Coronary Events in Older People with Frailty

Acute coronary syndromes (ACS) include ST-elevation myocardial infarct (STEMI), non-ST elevation MI (NSTEMI), and unstable angina. NSTEMI is more common than STEMI in older people. Like many conditions, there is a limited evidence base for treating ACS in people with frailty. Older people are underrepresented in clinical trials and are at greater risk of adverse outcomes.[1] This makes it even more important that we treat our patients as individuals.

Classical cardiac chest pain (i.e. crushing, central, radiation to neck, jaw, or left arm) is less common in older people with frailty. Alternative presentations include shortness of breath and/or clinical signs of heart failure. ECG changes include ST segment elevation/depression, T-wave changes, or left bundle branch block. But other changes are possible, and a normal ECG doesn't exclude ACS. An elevated serum concentration of troponin T suggests cardiac damage but can have an alternative explanation, e.g. pulmonary embolism or aortic dissection.

The modern management of STEMI mainly involves primary coronary intervention (PCI), provided it can be performed in a timely fashion. If not, then thrombolysis may be given, provided there are no contraindications. Some people with NSTEMI have PCI; otherwise, a blood-thinning medication, like fondaparinux, is given. The benefit of PCI is likely to be diminished or even lost for people with limited life expectancy and/or age over 90. Analgesia and oxygen, if saturation low, are other aspects of ACS management.

Antiplatelets

Antiplatelet drugs are for both the acute treatment and longer-term prevention of IHD. Bleeding risk is higher for older people with frailty. Dual antiplatelet use is recommended for most people with ACS. Typically, this is aspirin plus a $P2Y_{12}$ inhibitor (i.e. clopidogrel, prasugrel, or ticagrelor). This dual prescription is continued for 1 to 12 months, depending on the balance of bleeding and thrombotic event risks for the individual patient. Aspirin plus clopidogrel, rather than ticagrelor or prasugrel, may be more suitable for older people with frailty.[1] The limited available trial data in this population suggest lower risk of bleeding events with similar reduction in thrombotic events. Gastric protection with a proton pump inhibitor is usually recommended. After the period of dual antiplatelets, a single drug is continued (clopidogrel is probably a little more effective than aspirin for this).

Anticoagulants

People with ACS may already be prescribed an anticoagulant medication at the time of the event, e.g. a direct oral anticoagulant (DOAC) for pre-existing atrial fibrillation. In this scenario, the combination of a DOAC with a single antiplatelet agent, usually clopidogrel, appears to provide the best balance of preventing thrombotic events with a low risk of bleeding adverse events. The antiplatelet is usually added for a period of 6–12 months, depending on balance of risks.

Long-Term Management

Beneficial lifestyle changes, where relevant, include stopping smoking, increasing exercise, eating a balanced diet, and obtaining optimal weight. Statin medications reduce the risk of recurrent events. Although the evidence base is less clear in older people with frailty [see Case 19], the highest risk of recurrence occurs in the period just after an ACS event. In such a scenario, even people with a shorter life expectancy could benefit from treatment. Echocardiography is often performed to establish ejection fraction. People with symptomatic heart failure with reduced ejection fraction are likely to be considered for a range of other medications [see Case 19].

A discussion was had with Harold about the potential risks and benefits of medications for him. It was agreed that clopidogrel would be added to the aspirin he was already prescribed for a period of three months. After that time, his primary care team were asked to cease aspirin and continue clopidogrel alone. Because of the higher risk of bleeding, a proton pump inhibitor was also prescribed while he was taking dual antiplatelet therapy. He received a dose of fondaparinux for three days. His simvastatin, atenolol, and losartan were continued unchanged. His pulmonary oedema was resolved, and he was not prescribed any diuretic medication at the point of discharge.

Other Medication Changes

Harold has a long-term catheter. If there is no plan for a trial without catheter, using tamsulosin is unlikely to have any benefit. Tamsulosin could precipitate orthostatic hypotension. Why Harold is prescribed solifenacin is not clear from the history we have. If it was being used for urinary incontinence, then it is no longer beneficial with a catheter present. Some people with in-dwelling catheters experience bladder spasms. These are thought to be due to the bladder contracting on the catheter balloon. Theoretically, anticholinergic medications could reduce bladder contractions and, thus, reduce symptoms. We should find out if this was the rationale of prescribing for Harold. Anticholinergic medications, like solifenacin, can cause dry mouth and constipation. There is a more serious risk of cognitive decline with longer term exposure, with an estimated doubling of the risk of developing dementia.[2] We should ensure that any of our patients prescribed strong anticholinergic medications are aware of this risk when deciding about continuation versus deprescribing. Non-pharmacological ways to reduce bladder spasms, such as reducing the catheter balloon size, could be tried instead.

What about Harold?

Harold has mild to moderate frailty (CFS borderline 5 to 6). He was assessed by the physiotherapy team and was found to be able to mobilise at his pre-admission level, including doing the stairs. He felt that he was well supported at home and didn't want any extra help. He would like to return to hospital for treatment in the future should he develop health problems like pneumonia or another episode of ACS.

Key Points

- Although standardised protocols exist for the management of common conditions, like ACS, treatment often needs to be adjusted to suit individual patient needs and characteristics.
- Selecting the combination of antiplatelet/antithrombotic medications and their duration is a balance between the risk of recurrent thrombosis and bleeding complications for each person.

Further Reading

1. Byrne RA, Rossello X, Coughlan JJ, et al. 2023 ESC Guidelines for the management of acute coronary syndromes: developed by the task force on the management of acute coronary syndromes of the European Society of Cardiology (ESC). *Eur Heart J* 2023;44:3720–826. https://doi.org/10.1093/eurheartj/ehad191
2. Taylor-Rowan M, Edwards S, Noel-Storr AH, et al. Anticholinergic burden (prognostic factor) for prediction of dementia or cognitive decline in older adults with no known cognitive syndrome. *Cochrane Database Syst Rev* 2021;Issue 5. Art. No.: CD013540. https://doi.org/10.1002/14651858.CD013540.pub2

Roland

Roland is a 78-year-old man who had an unwitnessed fall while walking to his local shop. A passer-by took him home and notified his neighbours, who called for an ambulance. Roland recalls the fall but not the location where it occurred, stating it happened since he came into hospital. He said he had some preceding light-headedness, which he had also noticed on rapid standing since he had a stroke four months ago. Since his stroke, he has also noticed reduced vision on his right side. With his fall, he recalls tripping and landing on his left side but is unsure what he tripped over. There was no preceding shortness of breath or chest pain. He did not have loss of consciousness. He was not on the ground for long but required help from the passer-by to get to his feet. Once up, he had pain in the region of his left hip when putting weight through that leg. Since struggling back to his property with help, he has not been walking around. His partner, Sheila, has noticed some confusion since the stroke, but she does not feel that he is any more confused today compared to recently. He did not have any other symptoms.

Past Medical History

Left posterior circulation stroke four months ago—residual right homonymous hemianopia

Cognitive impairment (MOCA 9/30 during stroke admission)

Type 2 diabetes (T2DM) with retinopathy

Hypertension

Valvular heart disease (moderate aortic stenosis, moderate tricuspid regurgitation) last echocardiogram four months ago during stroke admission

Heart failure with mildly reduced ejection fraction (HFmrEF; EF 45%)

Chronic renal impairment

Previous DNACPR form completed and decision for a ward-based ceiling of care

Medication

Atorvastatin 80 mg od	Biphasic isophane insulin 14 units AM, 10 units PM
Bisoprolol 5 mg od	
Dapagliflozin 10 mg od	Clopidogrel 75 mg od
Finasteride 5 mg od	Eplerenone 25 mg od
Metformin MR 1g bd	Lansoprazole 30 mg od
Tamsulosin MR 400 mcg od	Sacubitril/valsartan 24/26 mg bd

 DOI: 10.1201/9781003582007-16

Social History

Roland lives alone in a house. He mobilises independently using a single walking stick, including doing the stairs in his property. Carers visit twice a day to assist with meal preparation only. He is independent with washing and dressing. He administers his own medications, including insulin. His partner, Sheila, lives several doors down from him, and they spend several hours together on most days.

Examination

Alertness is normal. He has an ejection systolic heart murmur. His JVP is not elevated, and there is no peripheral oedema. Chest is clear. Abdomen soft and non-tender. There is no external evidence of head injury, no cervical spine tenderness, and a normal range of neck motion. A graze to the left elbow has been covered with a dressing. The left hip is tender to palpate over the lateral aspect, but there is no shortening or external rotation. There is mild pain on straight leg raising and hip abduction on that side. Full range of eye movements, normal pupillary light reaction. Right homonymous hemianopia. Power normal in upper limbs and right leg, left leg limited by pain but able to move against gravity. Sensation is intact.

Six-Item Screener 3/6

4AT 2/12

BP was variable over the first two days of his admission, ranging between 110/60 and 171/80 mmHg, pulse 70 bpm regular, oxygen saturation 93% on air, temperature 36.4°C. Glucose in the range 5.0 to 8.9 mmol/L since admission.

Lying BP 125/66 mmHg and 126/55 mmHg after standing for one minute.

Weight 73.8 kg (body mass index 29 kg/m²)

Bowels open this morning (type 4 on the Bristol Stool Chart)

Investigations

Biochemistry	Value	Reference range	Haematology	Value	Reference range
Sodium	143	133–146 mmol/L	Haemoglobin	144	130–180 g/L
Potassium	4.3	3.5–5.3 mmol/L	MCV	91	82–100 fL
Urea	8.9	2.5–7.8 mmol/L	White cell count	13.1	4–11 10⁹/L
Creatinine	105	64–104 umol/L	Neutrophils	10.3	2–7.5 10⁹/L
C-reactive protein	2	< 5 mg/L	Platelets	279	140–400 10⁹/L

Liver blood tests and calcium normal

One month ago: urea 7.7, creatinine 119, Hb_{A1C} 53 mmol/mol

ECG—sinus rhythm 79 bpm

Why did Roland fall over?

How would you manage his blood pressure?

Regarding management of his diabetes, is his glucose appropriately controlled?

What is the appropriate management of his pelvic fracture?

What does his brain CT scan show?

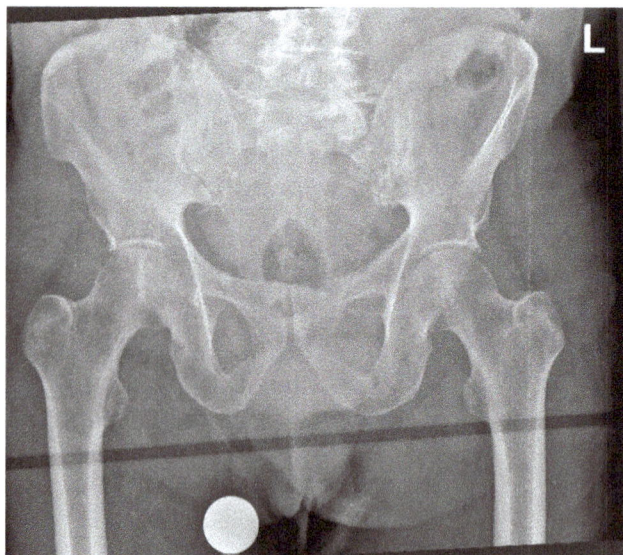

Figure 16.1 Pelvic X-ray showing a left superior pelvic ramus fracture.

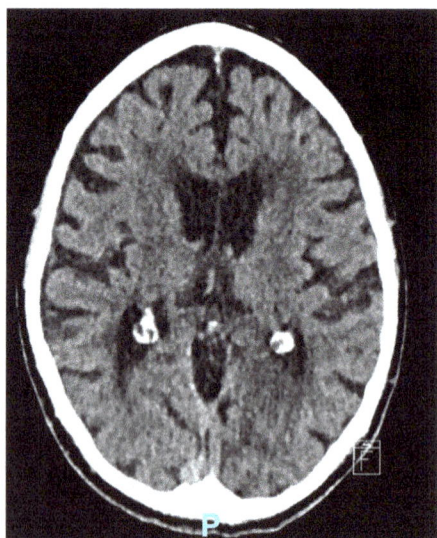

Figure 16.2 CT brain scan.

Why Did He Fall Over?

Roland reported light-headedness prior to his fall and sometimes when he stands quickly. This suggests there is an element of orthostatic hypotension (OH) in the mechanism of his fall. Although the lying and standing BP measurement during this admission did not detect a postural drop. This could be because his BP doesn't always dip when he stands, or maybe the technique used missed a brief dip between measurements. His supine BP has been variable during the admission. He takes several medications that could contribute to OH [see Case 11], i.e. bisoprolol, dapagliflozin, eplerenone, sacubitril/valsartan, and tamsulosin. He may have peripheral neuropathy caused by diabetes, and moderate aortic stenosis may also make his symptoms worse.

There are many other possible contributors to his fall. Notably since his stroke, he now has marked visual impairment, on a background of diabetic retinopathy, and is at risk of tripping over objects on his right side. His cognition has significantly declined. He may now forget about his physical impairments and move faster than would be advisable or neglect to use his walking stick. His blood sugars have been variable. Episodes of low blood glucose could also be a factor. Roland's situation and health is complex. A series of assessments and interventions (i.e. CGA) is likely to be required to optimise as many of these risk factors as possible.

Blood Pressure

Lower blood pressure is associated with reduced risk of future stroke. In the UK, guidelines recommend a target systolic BP consistently below 130 mmHg for most people who have had a stroke.[1] This recommendation was based on the results of randomised controlled trials. The mean age of participants in the relevant trials was much lower than Roland's age (around 64), and people with a complex mix of co-morbidities were rarely included. In geriatric medicine, it is hard to know how appropriate such recommendations are for the complex individual you are treating. In recognition of the lack of reliable trial data for people with frailty and co-morbidities, UK National Institute for Health and Care Excellence (NICE) guidelines for hypertension do not set a specific target BP for this group but instead simply suggest that clinical judgment is used.[2] In addition, Roland has presented following a fall, and he has symptoms suggesting OH. Episodes of low BP increase his risk of falling and injuring himself. The NICE hypertension guidelines also recommend measuring BP a minute after standing for people with suspected OH, and everyone aged over 80, and using the lower value obtained to formulate management decisions.[2] Either a stroke or a fall with a hip fracture could affect his long-term function and independence.

Roland's BP has been very variable while in hospital. He has a diagnosis of HFmrEF and is prescribed all the 'four pillars' [see Case 19], which could affect his BP. Aortic stenosis also complicates his management. BP varies in all of us, including in response to pain and anxiety. Cognitive impairment could increase distress around hospital admissions. There is no need to rush in to treat single high readings. A series of measurements, preferably taken when in a stable health condition, is required. In fact, some data suggest that intensifying anti-hypertensive medication during a non-cardiovascular hospital admission could result in harm.[3] Ambulatory BP monitoring, e.g. over 24 hours, can give additional information. Such tests can be requested after a patient has returned to their own home to get a data set more representative of their norm. During a hospital admission, the lowest BP is usually the most relevant. This could be a marker of illness, such as sepsis, and can help identify risk of falling.

There is always a balance of risks and benefits for medical treatments. Nobody knows what the future holds for Roland. Discussions about the clinical trial data and relative merits of each course of action are complex. They require a high degree of health literacy. Roland has cognitive impairment to complicate matters. His next of kin, which may be Sheila, can help contribute to discussions. If a decision is made to reduce the medication that he takes to lower BP, then stopping sacubitril/valsartan would be a reasonable place to start. Given his limited life expectancy, any prognostic benefit for heart failure or diabetic nephropathy is limited. Risks are elevated due to his OH and aortic stenosis.

Glucose Control

Tight glucose control is usually recommended for non- or mildly frail older people with T2DM, for example, Hb_{A1C} in the range 42 to 53 mmol/mol. Achieving such a target can reduce the risk of vascular complications, but this may take over ten years, which is less relevant for people with limited life expectancy. Tight glucose control increases the risk of hypoglycaemia, which can lead to multiple complications. In non-frail people, hypoglycaemia typically presents with sweating, tremor, and palpitations. People with frailty may present with neurological symptoms alone, which include slurred speech, falls, confusion, and seizures. Glucose is the brain's key energy source, yet the brain stores no glucose and cannot create it. Episodes of hypoglycaemia increase the risk of cognitive decline and dementia.[4]

Roland is vulnerable to hypoglycaemia because he lives alone and has cognitive impairment. His food intake may be variable. The key aim for Roland's diabetes management is preventing the osmotic symptoms of marked hyperglycaemia, i.e. polyuria, polydipsia, and weight loss. A much more lenient glucose target, perhaps Hb_{A1C} 64 to 75 mmol/mol, could achieve this with a lower risk of hypoglycaemia. As his latest Hb_{A1C} was 53 mmol/mol, and he has had glucose readings on the lower side while in hospital, a reduction in his insulin dose should be considered. Metformin and dapagliflozin can cause a little weight loss, but he is not underweight. Both these medications have lower risk of causing hypoglycaemia than insulin.

A complicating factor when adjusting diabetes medications during a hospital admission is that things could change once back at home. Oral intake could be reduced due to illness or increased due to easy access to meals. The type of foods could also change. Sometimes people choose more sugary things at home, sometimes people eat more in hospital, for example, chocolates and biscuits brought in by well-intentioned visitors. We also don't know about his adherence to prescribed medications at home, and it may be much higher during the admission. All these things emphasise the importance of good communication with community teams and follow-up.

Pelvic Fracture

The key components of managing pelvic fractures are providing adequate analgesia and mobilising as soon as possible. Pain control may require the use of opioids, which increase the risk of constipation. The co-prescription of a laxative should be considered at the time of opioid initiation. The physiotherapy team can help with advice about mobilisation and the use of walking aids or other equipment. This advice can then be utilised by other ward staff members to help the rehabilitation process. Roland's cognitive impairment may hinder recall of advice from one therapy session to another. This does not mean that he can't benefit from rehabilitation. It simply means that techniques will have to be adapted to work with his abilities.

Osteoporosis could be an underlying factor increasing Roland's risk of fracture. Some medications, including proton pump inhibitors, are associated with lower bone mineral density.[5] It is worth considering why Roland is prescribed lansoprazole, whether he is still getting symptomatic benefit, and if a dose reduction or withdrawal should be tried. Risk scores for osteoporosis (i.e. FRAX, QFracture) can be calculated using online tools. Bone mineral density can be measured by a DEXA scan to establish a diagnosis of osteoporosis. Standard treatment is a once-weekly oral bisphosphonate, often with a calcium and vitamin

D supplement. This potentially adds to Roland's medication burden. Oral bisphosphonates must be taken 30 minutes before any food or other medications in the morning, while sitting upright, and followed by a full glass of water. This can be challenging for people with frailty and cognitive impairment. These medications can't be placed within multi-dose dispensing boxes. An intravenous bisphosphonate, such as yearly zoledronate, avoids the need to take tablets orally but does require intravenous cannulation. Administration can lead to a flu-like illness for a few days afterwards.

Due to his combination of morbidities, and physical and cognitive frailty, Roland has limited life expectancy. Significant fracture risk reduction with bisphosphonates takes around 12 months to occur. Around 25 to 45 people with osteoporosis need to take a bisphosphonate for a period of two to three years to prevent a fracture.[6] Things are never black and white in geriatric medicine. Roland may feel that the associated therapeutic burden outweighs the chance of benefit for him. Reducing his risk of falls may be the most effective way to prevent future fractures.

CT Scan Discussion

Roland's brain CT scan shows generalised atrophy and small vessel ischaemic changes (Figure 16.3). There is also reduced attenuation in the left occipital lobe due to his old stroke.

What about Roland?

Roland has mild frailty (CFS 5) but has increased vulnerability due to his combination and physical and cognitive deficits. Sheila is concerned about Roland's memory loss and visual impairment, especially since his stroke. She has seen him struggle with simple tasks, such as making a cup of tea. She is unsure if he would manage between carer visits. She reports that his stairs are very steep and wonders if he will be able to safely use them much longer. The physiotherapy team can practice doing stairs while in hospital, but these may be dissimilar to

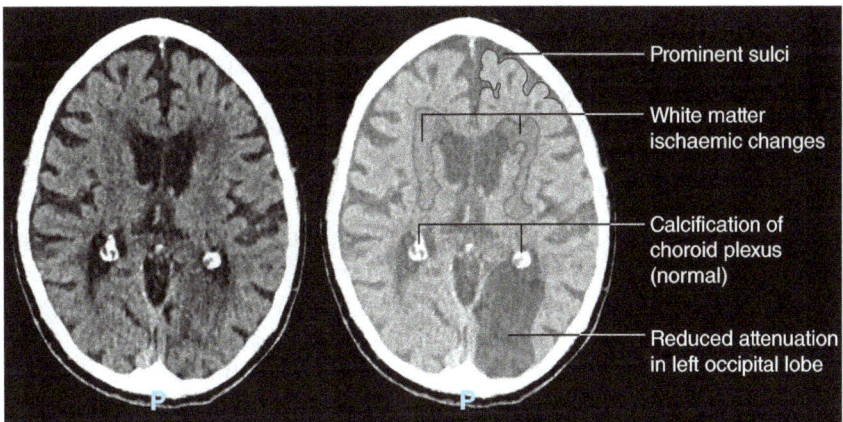

Figure 16.3 CT brain scan with annotation.

his own stairs. The occupational therapy (OT) team can perform functional assessments and could also arrange a home visit. This way, he could be observed using his own equipment, and stairs, in a familiar environment.

The OT discussed the option of downstairs living, but Sheila thinks that his family would prefer him to move into 24-hour care and are currently looking at local care homes. With Roland's permission, we need to identify who is his next of kin and establish the plan. We need to ask Roland what he would like to do. There may be a requirement to assess his mental capacity to decide his future place of residence [see Case 6]. Roland owns his current property. Maybe his next of kin has power of attorney to assist with his financial affairs. If Roland does return to his own property, he is likely to need an increase in his care package, both the frequency of visits and the assistance he receives. This could include helping him with his medications. Having some of his medications in a multi-dose administration aid could make it easier for the carers. Obviously, this would not include his insulin. The local district nursing team may be able to help safely manage his diabetes.

Key Points

- A single normal lying and standing BP measurement does not exclude OH.
- Increasing BP-lowering medications during an acute hospital admission may do more harm than good.
- More lenient targets for BP and glucose control are appropriate for older people with frailty.
- Around 25 to 45 people with osteoporosis need to take a bisphosphonate for a period of two to three years to prevent a fracture.

Further Reading

1. *National Stroke Guidelines*. 2023. www.strokeguideline.org/app/uploads/2023/04/National-Clinical-Guideline-for-Stroke–2023.pdf
2. National Institute for Health and Care Excellence. *Hypertension in Adults: Diagnosis and Management*. NG136. 2019. www.nice.org.uk/guidance/ng136
3. Anderson TS, Herzig SJ, Jing B, et al. Clinical outcomes of intensive inpatient blood pressure management in hospitalized older adults. *JAMA Intern Med* 2023;183:715–23. https://doi.org/10.1001/jamainternmed.2023.1667
4. Gómez-Guijarro MD, Álvarez-Bueno C, Saz-Lara A, et al. Association between severe hypoglycaemia and risk of dementia in patients with type 2 diabetes mellitus: a systematic review and meta-analysis. *Diabetes Metab Res Rev* 2023;39:e3610. https://doi.org/10.1002/dmrr.3610
5. Scottish Intercollegiate Guidelines Network. *Management of Osteoporosis and the Prevention of Fragility Fractures*. 2012. www.sign.ac.uk/our-guidelines/management-of-osteoporosis-and-the-prevention-of-fragility-fractures
6. Byun J, Jang S, Lee S, et al. The efficacy of bisphosphonates for prevention of osteoporotic fracture: an update meta-analysis. *J Bone Metable* 2017;24:37–49. https://doi.org/10.11005/jbm.2017.24.1.37

Case 17

Richard

Richard is an 85-year-old retired joiner. He was brought to hospital by ambulance because his carers were concerned about him being weaker and having more difficulty swallowing than usual. He said he had been feeling lethargic for a day or two and that his stroke side (the left side) was worse than usual. He also mentioned that his right foot ulcer was hurting. A prior discharge summary showed that he had been in hospital under the vascular surgeons a couple of months before this admission, and they had identified bilateral common femoral artery occlusions, which would be high risk for intervention, so he was 'to be managed conservatively'. He had seen his GP in the week leading up to admission, who had prescribed antibiotics for his right foot ulcer that was getting worse.

Past Medical History

Ischaemic heart disease—myocardial infarction 18 months ago
Right lacunar infarct stroke six years ago—some persistent left arm and leg weakness
Multiple previous right carotid TIAs, occluded right internal carotid artery
Peripheral vascular disease—bilateral common femoral artery occlusions
Benign prostatic hyperplasia

Medication

Atorvastatin 80 mg od	Clopidogrel 75 mg od
Codeine phosphate 30 mg as required	Colecalciferol 800 units od
Flucloxacillin 1 g qds for 14 days	Glyceryl trinitrate spray 400 mcg as
Lansoprazole 15 mg od	required
Propranolol 40 mg bd	Naftidrofuryl 100 mg tds
Tamsulosin MR 400 mcg od	Ramipril 2.5 mg od

Social History

Richard lives with his wife in a house that has a stairlift. He is independently mobile with a two-wheeled walking frame. He keeps one upstairs and one downstairs in the property. He rarely goes out of the house. Carers come in twice a day to help him get washed and dressed. His wife does most of the cooking and housework. Their daughter helps with shopping.

Examination

Heart sounds were normal, chest was clear, and there was no peripheral oedema. Abdominal examination was unremarkable. Power was reduced (4/5) in his left arm and leg. He had a deep ulcer between the 3rd and 4th toes of his right foot with some discharge. There was surrounding mottling of the skin. The right 1st toe was cold, and the whole right foot was cooler than the left.

Six-Item Screener 2/6

4AT 4/12

BP 164/57 mmHg, pulse 67 bpm, oxygen saturation 97% air, temperature 37.0°C, glucose 6.7 mmol/L

Investigations

Biochemistry	Value	Reference range	Haematology	Value	Reference range
Sodium	132	133–146 mmol/L	Haemoglobin	102	130–180 g/L
Potassium	5.1	3.5–5.3 mmol/L	MCV	91	82–100 fL
Urea	10.1	2.5–7.8 mmol/L	White cell count	14.1	4–11 10⁹/L
Creatinine	89	64–104 umol/L	Platelets	306	140–400 10⁹/L
C-reactive protein	68	< 5 mg/L			

Blood test six weeks ago: sodium 138, potassium 4.9, urea 10.3, creatinine 105

The admitting team felt that Richard had delirium and decompensation of his old stroke symptoms due to deterioration in his chronic ischaemic foot with possible superimposed infection. They discussed the situation with the local vascular surgical team, who identified that any surgical intervention would be very high risk. They did not think emergency revascularisation was feasible endovascularly. Their opinion was that he should be treated conservatively with antibiotics and fluids and that amputation could be considered if he deteriorated in the future.

Does Richard have an acutely ischaemic limb?
How could we have planned better with Richard?

Peripheral Vascular Disease

Critical limb-threatening ischaemia (CLTI) is a chronic condition (i.e. lasting more than two weeks) with some combination of symptoms, including rest pain, ulceration or gangrene, and infection. This is a progression from intermittent claudication in terms of symptoms and is usually caused by end-stage, systemic atherosclerosis. It is usefully differentiated from acute limb ischaemia (i.e. abrupt onset of painful, pale, pulseless, paralysed, paraesthetic, and perishingly cold limb) because this more frequently has a localised pathological cause and, consequently, different potential treatments.

Determinations around whether vascular surgeons offer an operative intervention for CLTI centre on whether the current clinical condition seems likely to lead to limb amputation. The Society for Vascular Surgery WIfI classification categorises combinations of symptoms and signs relating to the *Wound, Ischaemia,* and *foot Infection,* with worse conditions increasing the risk of amputation.[1] This then signals the potential value of revascularisation procedures (either surgical or endovascular) to attempt to salvage the limb. When a person with CLTI attends with worsening signs and symptoms, it alters their WIfI score and, consequently, their potential indication for surgery. This is a rather limb-centric view on risk/benefit. It is quite common for CLTI to deteriorate in the presence of significant illness, for example, through reduced tissue perfusion related to sepsis, dehydration, or heart failure. When this does develop in an older person with frailty who is hospitalised for another reason, it is often not a survivable situation, and operative intervention is neither possible nor desirable.

A study of various interventions (i.e. endovascular or surgical revascularisation, amputation, or conservative treatment) comparing those under or over 80 years showed that with successful revascularisation, the mortality of octogenarians was 32% at one year (compared with 17% of those < 80).[2] It also showed that amputation, compared to revascularisation, did not save lives. People tended to die early from issues related directly to the affected limb and later related to vascular disease in general, such as myocardial infarction or stroke. It is worth noting that revascularisation can be a temporising intervention with some people going on to have further revascularisation or amputation later if symptoms deteriorate again.

Guidelines for long-term management of CLTI recommend that all patients receive anti-platelet and cholesterol lowering treatments, also tight control of hypertension and diabetes. None of these measures have been shown to reduce the risk of revascularisation or amputation for CLTI. Their role is to reduce the risk of other cardiovascular conditions. As discussed in case 21, however, in the context of marked frailty and shortened life expectancy, a reduction in time for them to work and multiple competing causes of death could reduce their impact and make their prescription burdensome without significant benefit. Pain is ubiquitous in people with CLTI and causes distress and functional impairment. Adequate analgesia is an early patient-centred goal and is initiated with paracetamol and opioids as needed. Patients will often describe waking at night in bed and needing to let their leg hang over the side to relieve it. Some decide that sleeping in a chair is a better option, although this has obvious downsides.

In summary, CLTI indicates generalised atherosclerosis to the degree that there is insufficient blood getting to the peripheries. In a young and fit person, interventions can lead to short-term improvements, but consequences of the underlying cause remain significant. In older people with frailty, intervention is less likely to lead to survival or recovery to independence and may increase the symptom burden and medicalisation of late life. A shared decision-making approach is key.

Palliative Care and Advance Care Planning

Richard attended hospital with an acute deterioration in his foot pain, which had led to previous admissions and caused frequent severe symptoms over several months. It was clear that his advanced generalised vascular disease was likely to cause deterioration and death. It was also noted that his bilateral common femoral artery occlusions had been deemed 'not suitable for endovascular intervention' and that no one thought an open surgical approach was wise.

Significant illness with a potential surgical cure in older people with frailty is a more complicated area than it used to be even a few years ago. With improved surgical and peri-operative techniques and practices alongside a more multi-disciplinary approach to care, the chance of survival has increased across various specialties. Surgeons have operated on older and frailer patients in both elective and emergency settings. The risk associated with any elective procedure is far lower than its emergency counterpart, yet we see people being told they cannot have an elective procedure based on their physiological reserve only to have the same procedure (or a bigger one) in an emergency. This is because in the elective setting, the concern is that the operation might make things worse for the person. Yet in the emergency setting, things are already much worse, and the conception is of life-saving surgery rather than life-enhancing.

What has become increasingly clear, however, is that the concerns of people in surgical crises are not so much around dying (they know death is likely), but rather, they are concerned about ending up cognitively impaired, a burden to others, or losing their independence. Patients want to discuss what they might realistically expect to happen if they were to undergo surgery or not.[3,4] The shared decision of whether to use operative management is much more a balance of longer-term life goals alongside the journey they are likely to go through to try to get there. A study of a teaching programme delivered by palliative care services to surgical services raised the idea that death was not the worst outcome for everyone. Perhaps survival in a very dependent way would be considered worse than death by some people. Or that death very soon after a surgical attempt to save life might be preferable to a long and difficult recovery period in hospital ending in death.

Of course, for many older people living with frailty, the idea of going through a large operation and the ordeal of trying to recover and regain some semblance of real life seems unwise and undesirable. Conservative, comfort-based care giving them a chance to spend what life they have left unfettered by all the trappings of modern medicine is a choice they might make. So the paradigm may be less one of long-term condition management or curative treatment and more one of slow and unpredictable palliation.

What about Richard?

Richard has moderate frailty (CFS 6). For him, there seems to have been a missed opportunity to undertake advance care planning. His symptoms were caused by an untreatable, deteriorating surgical condition. He was struggling with significant pain and worsening ulceration of his foot. There was a relatively high chance of wet gangrene leading to very rapid deterioration and death. This was a palliative situation, proactive care might have reduced his symptom burden, and he could also have been able to make choices about where he wanted to be cared for at the end of his life. In the event, neither he nor his wife wanted him to go through an emergency limb amputation. His hospital care was primarily coordinated by the palliative care team. Severe pain and the release of inflammatory mediators from dying tissue caused significant delirium, which was challenging to manage. His family were allowed open visiting and were offered spiritual and emotional support. He died in the hospital.

Key Points

- Critical limb-threatening ischaemia is a very serious condition with associated high mortality. Interventions are aimed at limb salvage, symptom relief, and control of infection.
- Decisions about whether to undertake surgical treatments on older people with frailty require careful shared decision-making conversations centred on realistic outcomes and recovery expectations.
- When a burdensome condition is worsening and considered untreatable, advance care planning options, including wishes around late life and death, should be openly discussed.

Further Reading

1. Mills JL, Conte MS, Armstrong DG, et al. The Society for Vascular Surgery lower extremity threatened limb classification system: risk stratification based on Wound, Ischemia, and foot Infection (WIfI). *J Vasc Surg* 2014;59:220–34. https://doi.org/10.1016/j.jvs.2013.08.003

2. Wübbeke LF, Naves CCLM, Daemen JHC, et al. Mortality and major amputation after revascularisation in octogenarians versus non-octogenarians with chronic limb threatening ischaemia: a systematic review and meta-analysis. *Eur J Vasc Endovasc Surg* 2020;60:231–41. https://doi.org/10.1016/j.ejvs.2020.04.027

3. Taylor LJ, Nabozny MJ, Steffens NM, et al. A framework to improve surgeon communication in high-stakes surgical decisions: best case/worst case. *JAMA Surg* 2017;152:531–8. https://doi.org/10.1001/jamasurg.2016.5674

4. Law J, Welch C, Javanmard-Emamghissi H, et al. Decision-making for older patients undergoing emergency laparotomy: defining patient and clinician values and priorities. *Colorectal Dis* 2020;22:1694–703. https://doi.org/10.1111/codi.15165

Case 18

Lilian

Lilian is a 93-year-old retired shopkeeper who presented to hospital after a fall at home. Her main complaint in the emergency department is abdominal pain, which started yesterday. She has not had any nausea or vomiting. She often gets constipated. Her bowels were open yesterday, but she passed only a small amount of hard stool. She has not passed any urine today. She has also had a mild cough and shortness of breath, which has been slowly worsening over many weeks.

Past Medical History

Atrial fibrillation (AF)—on rivaroxaban
Cardiac pacemaker (slow AF and falls)
T2DM
Hypertension
Diverticular disease
Bullous pemphigoid (treated with steroids eight years ago)

Medication

Alendronate 70 mg weekly started eight years ago	Calcium and vitamin D one tablet bd
Codeine 15 mg as required	Ferrous sulfate 200 mg od
Fexofenadine 180 mg od	Furosemide 80 mg am and 40 mg noon
Losartan 100 mg od	Macrogol as required
Omeprazole 10 od	Paracetamol 500 mg as required
Rivaroxaban 15 mg od	Senna 7.5 mg as required

Social History

Lilian lives alone in a house with a stairlift. She has a two-wheeled walking frame both upstairs and downstairs. Sometimes she doesn't use the frame and holds on to the furniture in her property instead. She can wash and dress herself, but it takes her a long time. Her daughter helps with shopping and some housework.

 DOI: 10.1201/9781003582007-18

Examination

She appears comfortable while lying in bed. The pacemaker is noted on her left upper chest. There is mild wheeze in her chest. Heart sounds are normal. JVP not elevated. Her abdomen looks mildly distended and is soft but tender over the left side. No masses or lumps are detected. Bowel sounds are present. There is some mild bilateral leg oedema.

Six-Item Screener 5/6

4AT 1/12

BP 113/67 mmHg, pulse 65 bpm, oxygen saturation 93% on air, temperature 35.6°C

Bladder scan 489 mls

Investigations

Biochemistry	Value	Reference range	Haematology	Value	Reference range
Sodium	131	133–146 mmol/L	Haemoglobin	93	115–165 g/L
Potassium	4.3	3.5–5.3 mmol/L	MCV	83	82–100 fL
Urea	10.2	2.5–7.8 mmol/L	White cell count	8.3	4–11 10^9/L
Creatinine	175	49–90 umol/L	Platelets	258	140–400 10^9/L
C-reactive protein	6	< 5 mg/L	Ferritin	25.7	12–250 µg/L
Albumin	35	35–50 g/L	Vitamin B_{12}	478	150–1000 ng/L
Adjusted calcium	2.35	2.2–2.6 mmol/L	Folate	4.0	2–18.8 ug/L

Blood tests three months ago: sodium 134, urea 8.3, creatinine 119

Why has Lilian developed urinary retention?

Why might she be constipated, and how would you treat it?

Urinary Retention

Urinary retention can develop due to a neurological impairment of the bladder nerves or a physical blockage to the bladder outflow tract. Neurological impairment can be caused by anticholinergic medications, peripheral neuropathy (e.g. diabetes), and sometimes a spinal cord problem (e.g. cauda equina syndrome). Neurological causes are more likely to be painless and present with a continual dribbling of small volumes of urine. In men, bladder outflow tract obstruction often occurs secondary to benign prostatic hyperplasia (BPH). Constipation is the common cause affecting both men and women. The large bowel and urethra pass through the pelvis. Enlargement of either the bowel or bladder can reduce the available space. This is shown in Figure 18.3. Outflow tract obstruction is often very painful but can present as hypoactive delirium without obvious pain.

Clinical history is likely to give clues to the underlying problem. Physical examination may reveal an enlarged bladder. Rectal examination may demonstrate faecal impaction

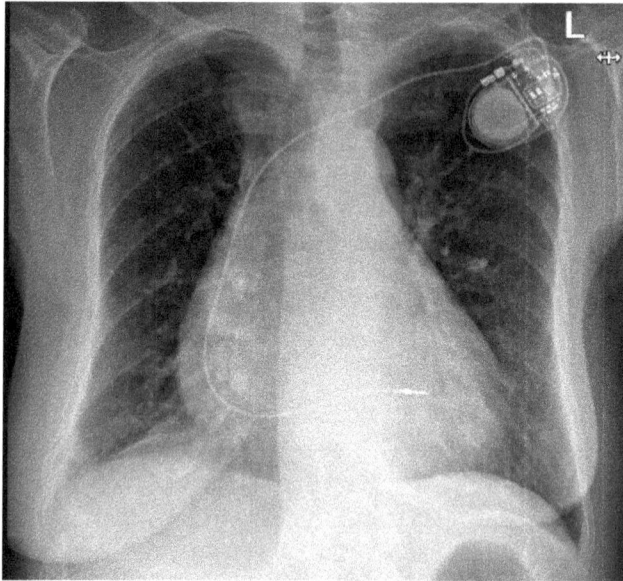

Figure 18.1 Chest X-ray showing single-lead pacemaker and an enlarged cardiac silhouette.

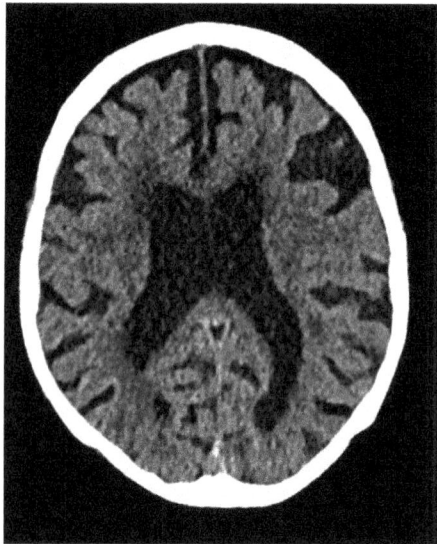

Figure 18.2 CT head showing generalised atrophy and small vessel ischaemic changes.

or prostatic enlargement. A bladder scan is also helpful. For Lilian, her history suggests underlying constipation. Her bladder scan confirms urinary retention (489 ml). Older people don't always empty their bladder as completely as younger people, but the post-void volume should still be < 200 ml. Although there is no absolute cutoff above which a post-void residual volume necessitates a urinary catheter, a rough guide would be > 500 ml and/or symptomatic

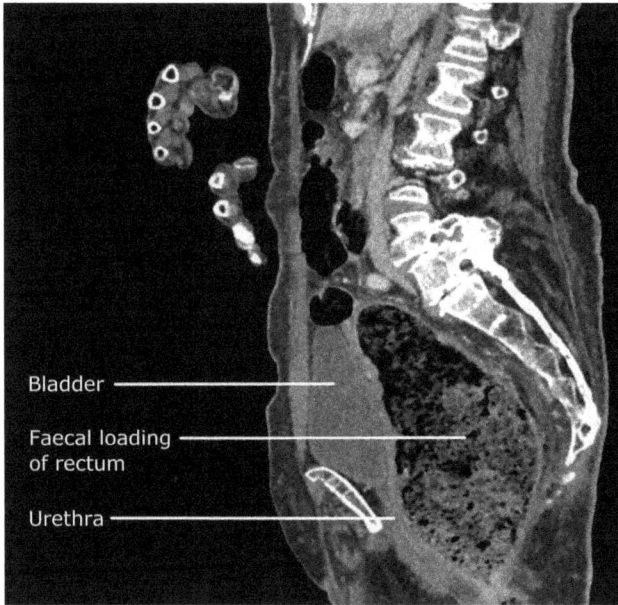

Figure 18.3 CT image showing that faecal impaction can cause compression of the bladder outflow tract.

(e.g. discomfort). For Lilian, she has presented with abdominal pain, which may be partly related to urinary retention. Also, emptying her bladder may make treating her constipation easier. The standard first management step for retention is catheterisation to relieve the obstruction. It is usually possible to remove the catheter once the cause of retention has been identified and corrected.

Urinary Catheters

In geriatric medicine, the usual indication for urethral catheter insertion is urinary retention. Sometimes catheters are used to monitor fluid balance in the context of severe acute illness. Occasionally, they are used for people with urinary incontinence, where there is a need to protect compromised skin or a healing pressure ulcer. Catheters can be appropriate in other situations. For example, a man who must get up every 30 minutes overnight due to BPH, leading to exhaustion, while awaiting definitive prostate treatment.

The main adverse effect of catheters is the increased risk of urinary tract infection. They also affect sexual function. There is also the need to carry a bag of urine around. Some people find catheters very difficult to tolerate, possibly resulting in pulling them out. Catheterisation also increases the risk of delirium. General rules of geriatrics are to avoid catheterisation whenever possible and remove any catheter as soon as you can. To achieve this latter goal, it is important to establish when a catheter was inserted and the indication (including residual volume drained if inserted for retention), with clear documentation.

If the catheter was inserted for retention, then ensure the patient's bowels are emptying and potential culprit medications (e.g. anticholinergics) are minimised before withdrawal. Because of BPH, men are at higher risk of complete obstruction of the urinary tract.

117

Longstanding impaired emptying leads to enlargement of the bladder. The normal upper limit of bladder volume is around 700 ml for most people. The residual volume of urine drained directly after catheterisation should be noted. When residual urine volumes exceed 1 litre, there is a high probability of chronic urinary retention. In this scenario, unless remedial action is taken, removing the catheter will probably simply lead to recurrent urinary retention. For men with BPH, remedial action is likely to involve starting a new medication or having a surgical procedure. Long-term catheter use is sometimes the best option. People with impaired physical or cognitive function may require assistance to manage a catheter. When a patient is discharged with a catheter, ensure that they have any necessary support (consider district nursing input) and communicate any plans to the primary care team.

Constipation

Although constipation has a wide range of potential causes, including bowel diseases, in geriatric medicine, the classic triad is a combination of dehydration, immobility, and medication adverse effects (see Figure 18.4). Occasionally, other medical problems not directly related to the bowel can cause constipation, examples include hypercalcaemia and hypothyroidism.

In healthcare settings, the detection of constipation is aided by recording bowel activity and stool appearance. The Bristol Stool Chart is used to rate bowel motions, based on water content, from 1 (more solid) to 7 (more liquid). Infrequent bowel motions and passing stool types 1 or 2 suggest constipation. Sometimes faecal impaction can cause liquid stool to pass around the obstruction. This scenario is termed 'overflow diarrhoea' and can, paradoxically, result in people who are severely constipated passing type 7 stools. In this scenario, there is likely to be a history of absent bowel motions for several days before the diarrhoea develops, and there may be a palpable faecal mass on abdominal examination.

Untreated constipation can lead to a range of problems, including faecal impaction, urinary retention, functional decline, and delirium. Non-pharmacological approaches include rehydration, deprescribing potentially constipating medications, and optimising mobility. Ideally, patients will get to a standard toilet rather than attempt to do a poo on a bedpan or on a commode behind a curtain on a busy ward. Laxative medications are also

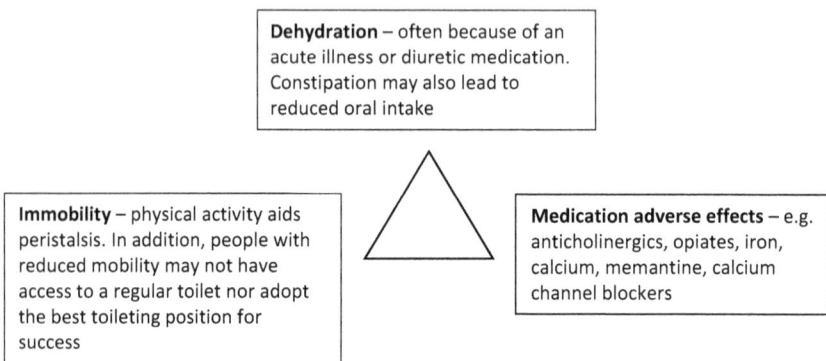

Dehydration – often because of an acute illness or diuretic medication. Constipation may also lead to reduced oral intake

Immobility – physical activity aids peristalsis. In addition, people with reduced mobility may not have access to a regular toilet nor adopt the best toileting position for success

Medication adverse effects – e.g. anticholinergics, opiates, iron, calcium, memantine, calcium channel blockers

Figure 18.4 Common precipitants of constipation for older people with frailty.

usually required. The prophylactic prescription of a laxative should be considered when starting high-risk medications, such as opioids.

Senna or bisacodyl are stimulant laxatives, which are often effective and well tolerated. They only require taking tablets, which means they are suitable for some people with reduced oral intake. Macrogol is an osmotic laxative. It is effective but requires taking a reasonable volume of liquid and may not be suitable for people with very limited oral intake. Thickening agents cannot be added to macrogol, which is relevant to some people taking a modified diet. Lactulose is an osmotic laxative that only requires taking a smaller volume of liquid but is probably less effective. Fibre-containing laxatives are unsuitable for frail older people because they need to be taken with large volumes of fluid or could worsen the constipation. Sodium docusate is described as a stool softener but has evidence of inefficacy and should not be prescribed. Enemas are useful for people with limited oral intake or for the resolution of faecal impaction.

What about Lilian?

The causative factors for Lilian developing constipation included all three of dehydration, reduced mobility, and medication adverse effects. Through discussion of the risks and benefits of the various options with Lilian, a management plan was formed.

Codeine, ferrous sulfate, and the calcium/vitamin D supplement were discontinued. Her pain was adequately controlled with paracetamol alone. She was given an intravenous iron supplementation to avoid the need to take the constipating tablets. She had been prescribed calcium and vitamin D supplements along with alendronate since she received a course of oral steroids for bullous pemphigoid eight years ago. As she had not received any steroids in the last few years, it was agreed that she could now discontinue alendronate, calcium, and vitamin D [see Case 4]. The losartan she had been taking was also deprescribed because her BP was on the lower side, she had presented with a fall, and it was unlikely to provide any prognostic benefit for her. The fexofenadine was for itch related to her bullous pemphigoid, and she used it sparingly but found it useful. This has the lowest anticholinergic burden of the common antihistamines so was unlikely to contribute to her presenting symptoms. It was discussed with her whether she should continue rivaroxaban. She had fallen over and had anaemia due to iron deficiency. One of Lilian's key fears was having a stroke and becoming more functionally impaired. For this reason, it was agreed that she would remain on rivaroxaban.

Her initial blood tests showed her urea was elevated. She was prescribed furosemide and had some leg oedema. Her JVP was not elevated, and her chest X-ray did not show pulmonary oedema. There are several potential causes of leg oedema [see Case 4]. Due to the threshold effect of loop diuretics, the variable 80/40 dosing of furosemide doesn't make sense.[1] The lowest effective dose should be prescribed each time. Lilians's diuretic was initially withheld. Her leg oedema worsened while off furosemide. She was discharged home on a reduced dose of 40 mg od. At this dose, her leg oedema was controlled, and blood tests showed her urea had returned to within the normal range.

With help from the physiotherapy team, her mobility was optimised during her admission. These steps, along with receiving senna and macrogol regularly, resolved her constipation. Her urinary catheter was successfully removed prior to discharge. The shortness of breath and cough that were reported at the time of her admission resolved without any cause being identified. She was assessed by the occupational therapy and social work teams, and a care package was provided twice a day to help her with washing and dressing. She was followed up by the virtual ward team, who rechecked her blood tests and assessed for worsening oedema or recurrent constipation in the week following her return home from hospital.

Key Points

- Urinary retention and constipation often co-exist.
- Look for dehydration, immobility, and medication adverse effects when assessing older people with frailty and constipation.
- The standard geriatric approach to urinary catheters is to avoid them whenever possible and remove them as soon as you can.

Further Reading

1. Anisman SD, Erickson SB, Morden NE. How to prescribe loop diuretics in oedema. *BMJ* 2019;364. https://doi.org/10.1136/bmj.l359

Case 19

Abdul

Abdul is an 85-year-old retired railway worker who presented to hospital after a fall. There had been a general decline in his health over the past month, with lack of appetite and weight loss. He had had multiple falls in the last week. He had fallen the evening prior to admission, hurting his right shoulder. He had fallen on the preceding weekend and bumped his head, sustaining a laceration to his scalp. Understandably, his family were increasingly concerned. Around 11 on the morning of arrival, he had had another fall but didn't injure himself. His wife had called his daughter to make her aware of recent events, and they agreed that it was time to call an ambulance. Abdul said he simply fell to the ground without any warning symptoms. He did not report any loss of consciousness with the falls. There had not been any recent vomiting, visual disturbance, or change in cognition.

Past Medical History

Heart failure with reduced ejection fraction (HFrEF)
Atrial fibrillation
Ischaemic heart disease (IHD)—myocardial infarction and coronary artery bypass grafts 12 years ago
Peripheral vascular disease with angioplasty of superficial femoral artery
Gallbladder calculus
Gastritis/duodenitis
Gout

Medication

Allopurinol 200 mg od	Apixaban 2.5 mg bd
Atorvastatin 80 mg od	Carvedilol 3.125 mg bd
Codeine 15 mg as required	Dapagliflozin 10 mg od
Glyceryl trinitrate 400 mcg sublingual as required	Ibuprofen 10% gel
	Paracetamol 500 mg as required
Omeprazole 20 mg gastro-resistant od	Spironolactone 25 mg od
Sacubitril 24 mg/valsartan 26 mg bd	

Social History

Abdul lives with his wife in a terraced house. He furniture walks around the property and doesn't go out alone anymore. He finds the stairs a struggle. The house has toilets both

DOI: 10.1201/9781003582007-19

upstairs and downstairs. His family provides support with some aspects of his personal care, but he has no formal care package. He quit smoking after his heart attack 12 years ago and has never drunk alcohol.

Examination

Adbul is alert. There are superficial abrasions on his forehead and a healing laceration to the right side of his scalp. His right shoulder is swollen and mildly bruised over the humeral head, but he can move through a normal range with only mild discomfort. No other injuries or bruises were seen elsewhere.

His pulse is irregular. Heart sounds normal. Chest clear. Abdomen soft and non-tender. Bowel sounds normal. He is not tender over the pelvic bones. His hips move through a good range of motion without pain. There is no neck tenderness on palpation. No focal neurological deficit is detected.

4AT 0/12

Six-Item Screener 5/6

BP 121/57, pulse 82 bpm, oxygen saturation 100% on air, temperature 36.5°C, weight 55.7kg, glucose 5.3 mmol/L

Lying BP 137/65 mmHg and one minute after standing 102/57 mmHg

Investigations

Biochemistry	Value	Reference range	Haematology	Value	Reference range
Sodium	136	133–146 mmol/L	Haemoglobin	115	130–180 g/L
Potassium	4.6	3.5–5.3 mmol/L	MCV	98	82–100 fL
Urea	9.9	2.5–7.8 mmol/L	White cell count	8.2	4–11 10⁹/L
Creatinine	74	64–104 umol/L	Platelets	197	140–400 10⁹/L
C-reactive protein	14	< 5 mg/L			
Albumin	35	35–50 g/L	Ferritin	153	12–250 ug/L
Adjusted calcium	2.28	2.2–2.6 mmol/L	Vitamin B_{12}	177	150–1000 ng/L
TSH	1.8	0.3–4.5 mIU/L	Folate	5.3	2–18.8 ug/L
Uric acid	209	200–430 µmol/L			

Liver blood tests normal. Urea 4.4 three months ago.
ECG—atrial fibrillation, 87 beats per minute, no ischaemic changes

Echocardiogram a month ago: mildly dilated left ventricle with eccentric hypertrophy and severely impaired systolic function, estimated EF 30 to 35%. Normal right ventricular size with mildly impaired function. Bi-atrial dilation. No significant heart valve lesions.

What is the optimal management of Abdul's heart failure?
Why is he falling over?
What are the likely risks and benefits of statins for Abdul?
Would you change any other medications?

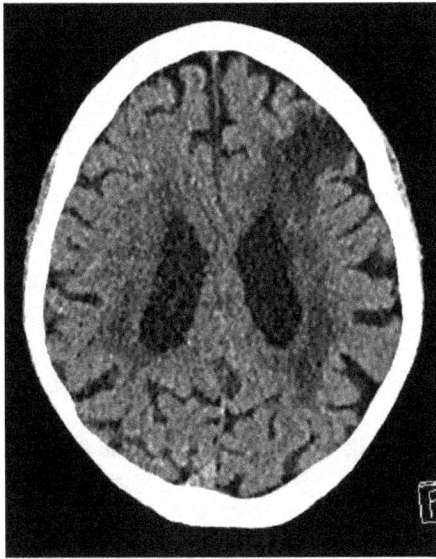

Figure 19.1 CT head showing extensive small vessel ischaemic changes and an old left frontal lobe stroke.

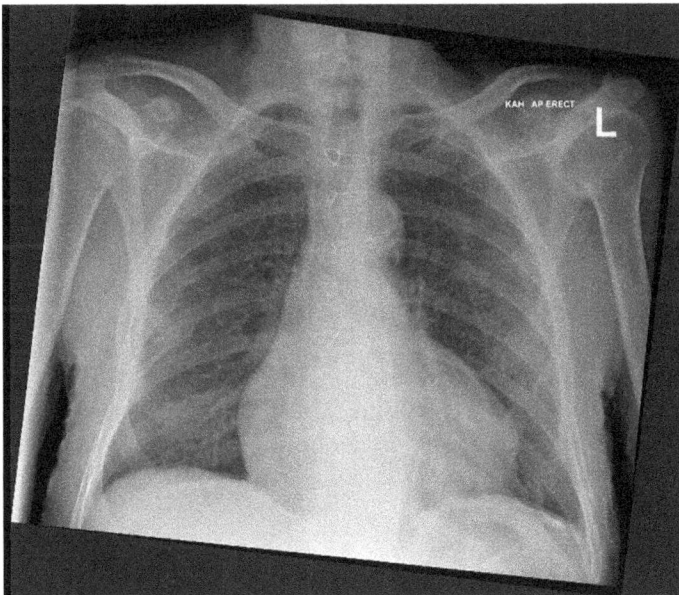

Figure 19.2 Chest X-ray showing sternal wires from previous heart surgery and small pleural plaques on his diaphragm, but the lung fields appear clear.

What is the Optimal Management of his Heart Failure?

Abdul has a diagnosis of heart failure with reduced ejection fraction (HFrEF), i.e. EF 40% or below. The modern management of heart failure has progressed over recent years. Current guidelines recommend that all patients with HFrEF should be considered for a combination of four medications,[1] which are an ACE inhibitor (ACEi) or angiotensin receptor blocker and neprilysin inhibitor combination (ARNI), a beta blocker (BB), a mineralocorticoid receptor antagonist (MRA), and a sodium-glucose co-transporter 2 inhibitor (SGLT2i). These are usually prescribed in addition to a loop diuretic for symptom control, often adding five medications to their list.

The rationale for these recommendations is based on the outcomes of clinical trials that showed a benefit. But these trials recruited carefully selected people.[2] For example, the average age of people was typically in the range 61 to 67 years, and people with significant co-morbidities were often excluded. Because frailty is a state of increased vulnerability, including susceptibility to adverse drug reactions, having few people with frailty in the clinical trials could mask the risk of harm. For each medication, the number needed to treat to prevent one adverse cardiovascular event typically ranged from 19 to 31 over trial durations of 1.3 to 2.2 years. Thus, most people prescribed these medications will not avoid an adverse event in any given year.

Abdul is currently prescribed all four recommended medications for HFrEF (BB, ARNI, MRA, SGLT2i). Dapagliflozin, an SGLT2i, is discussed in more detail in Case 30. Sacubitril/valsartan is an ARNI. Sacubitril is the neprilysin inhibitor component that blocks the breakdown of natriuretic compounds, thus adding a mild diuretic effect to an angiotensin receptor blocker. Potential risks include hypotension.

Around 40% of people aged over 85 with heart failure will die in the next year.[3] Abdul's recent health decline, falls, and degree of frailty (CFS 6) suggest that his prognosis may be worse than average for his age. We must discuss what is important to him. Clinical trials suggest continuing his medications for HFrEF would improve his prognosis. But the trials excluded people like Abdul. Risks of the medications include hypotension, or worsening OH, and thus making him more likely to fall over. This could also have a major impact, possibly threatening his ability to mobilise independently or risk injury, such as a broken hip.

On examination, he does not appear fluid overloaded, and his blood tests show an elevated urea, suggesting a degree of dehydration. He does not require a loop diuretic for heart failure symptom control. If the key goal is to reduce the risk of falling, then reducing medications most likely to lower BP should be considered. The ARNI is likely to have the biggest effect on BP. The SGLT2i could also lower his BP to a smaller extent. His blood tests suggest mild dehydration, which may be made worse by the MRA. The BB is less likely to cause hypotension but could still contribute to OH. Although it may have an additional benefit of controlling his heart rate with AF.

Statins

Statins are 3-hydroxy-3-methylglutaryl coenzyme A inhibitors that reduce cholesterol synthesis and have been proven to be effective at reducing cardiovascular disease in selected populations. In the UK, commonly prescribed statins include atorvastatin, rosuvastatin, and simvastatin. A meta-analysis of key trials found that statins were effective for secondary vascular prevention for people aged over 75, but the effect size was smaller in this age group than any other.[4] The NNT per year per mmol/L low density lipoprotein cholesterol reduction was 125. Very few people aged over 80 were recruited into these trials. The concept of 'competing cause of death' is relevant to people with multi-morbidity. A greater risk of dying from non-cardiovascular diseases reduces the potential survival advantage of avoiding a cardiovascular death.[5] Although statins can reduce the incidence of heart failure for people with IHD, the evidence for benefit for people with established heart failure is less strong.[6]

Statin intolerance affects some people. The actual incidence is unclear. The proportion of people affected in randomised clinical trials was much lower than that reported in observational studies. Statins can cause muscle symptoms. Possible presentations range from myalgia (i.e. muscle pain without a serum creatine kinase rise), to myositis (i.e. muscle pain plus a creatine kinase rise), to rhabdomyolysis (i.e. renal failure due to massive muscle breakdown, which is very rare). The risk of statin intolerance is increased in older age and with higher statin doses.[7] Minor muscle symptoms could have a significant functional impact for someone with frailty and sarcopenia. The lowest available dose of atorvastatin (10 mg) has over two-thirds of the lipid-lowering effect of the maximum dose (80 mg).[8] Reducing statin dose presents a possible alternative to either continuation or deprescribing.

What about Abdul?

Abdul's description of his falls does not give a clear causative mechanism. Several factors are likely to be contributing. We know that he has gait and balance impairment, as evidenced by furniture walking. We have also detected a postural drop in his blood pressure. There may also be environmental hazards in his home. Looking at his medications and assessments by the physiotherapy and occupational therapy teams are good places to start.

Adbul's main goal was to be able to return home and spend as much time as possible with his wife and family. He was adamant that he never wanted to live in a care home. He wanted to reduce his risk of falling to enable him to get around his property avoiding any broken bones. To reduce his risk of OH, his ARNI and MRA were discontinued. He wanted to remain on apixaban to reduce his risk of future stroke and loss of independence. Given his low muscle mass and declining mobility, it was agreed that his atorvastatin dose would be reduced from 80 mg to 10 mg daily. This seemed a reasonable compromise because he had a history of vascular disease. He had not had a flare of gout for many years. Because his urate was well below the therapeutic target of < 360 μmol/L, his allopurinol dose was reduced to 100 mg daily to lower his medication burden.

The physiotherapy team provided Adbul with two-wheeled walking frames for upstairs and downstairs in his property. They practiced mobility, including on the stairs. The occupational therapy team arranged for a second banister rail to be fitted at home. Adbul's family also discussed getting a stairlift installed in the future. A home visit was completed. Advice was given regarding reducing home hazards, such as loose rugs and inadequate lighting over the stairs. A raised toilet seat and bed lever were provided. Grab rails were fitted around his shower. Abdul did not want to consider having a care package, and his family were keen to continue supporting him at home.

Key Points

- People with frailty are at greater risk of harm from medications, and reduced life expectancy may attenuate potential benefits.
- Guidelines for single conditions need tailoring to suit an individual with frailty and multi-morbidity to ensure benefits exceed harms and are compatible with their goals.
- Shared decision-making can help to personalise care.

Further Reading

1. 2021 ESC Guidelines for the diagnosis and treatment of acute and chronic heart failure. *Eur Heart J* 2021;42:3599–726. https://doi.org/10.1093/eurheartj/ehab368

2. Woodford HJ, McKenzie D, Pollock LM. Appropriate management of heart failure in older people with frailty. *BMJ* 2024;387:e078188. https://doi.org/10.1136/bmj-2023–078188

3. Taylor CJ, Ordóñez-Mena JM, Roalfe AK, et al. Trends in survival after a diagnosis of heart failure in the United Kingdom 2000–2017: population based cohort study. *BMJ* 2019;364:l223. https://doi.org/10.1136/bmj.l223

4. Cholesterol Treatment Trialists' Collaboration. Efficacy and safety of statin therapy in older people: a meta-analysis of individual participant data from 28 randomised controlled trials. *Lancet* 2019;393:407–15. https://doi.org/10.1016/S0140–6736(18)31942–1

5. Kim CA, Kim DH. Statins provide less benefit in populations with high noncardiovascular mortality risk: meta-regression of randomized controlled trials. *J Am Geriatr Soc* 2015;63:1413–9. https://doi.org/10.1111/jgs.13476

6. Lee MMY, Sattar N, McMurray JJV, et al. Statins in the prevention and treatment of heart failure: a review of the evidence. *Curr Atherosclerosis Rep* 2019;21:41. https://doi.org/10.1007/s11883-019-0800-z

7. Bytyçi I, Penson PE, Mikhailidis DP, et al. Prevalence of statin intolerance: a meta-analysis. *Eur Heart J* 2022;43:3213–23. https://doi.org/10.1093/eurheartj/ehac015

8. Law MR, Wald NJ, Rudnicka AR. Quantifying effect of statins on low density lipoprotein cholesterol, ischaemic heart disease, and stroke: systematic review and meta-analysis. *BMJ* 2003;326:1423. https://doi.org/10.1136/bmj.326.7404.1423

Case 20

Elizabeth

Elizabeth is a 79-year-old retired optometrist who was admitted after a fall. She described tripping over one of her slippers that evening. Afterwards, she noticed pain in her right hip. Consequently, she was struggling to mobilise. Her two daughters came with her to the emergency department and were very concerned about their mother. They had found her on the floor in her home. They report that her mobility had declined rapidly over the past two weeks with increasing confusion and visual hallucinations. Her gait was described as looking like her feet were sticking to the floor. She had told her daughters that she had seen spiders on her walls when they visited. She had also fallen a week ago but without apparent injury. Her daughters now feel that she is unsafe at home. Apart from right hip pain, Elizabeth did not currently report any other symptoms.

Past Medical History

Possible Parkinson's disease—'not a candidate for medications' recorded in clinic letter last year
'Organic hallucinosis' diagnosed by the psychiatry team two years ago
Vertigo
Constipation
Ischaemic heart disease—myocardial infarct six years ago
Hypertension
Orthostatic hypotension (OH)

Medication

Aspirin 75 mg od	Atorvastatin 40 mg od
Bisoprolol 7.5 mg od	Glyceryl trinitrate 400 mcg sublingual as
Lansoprazole 15 mg od	required
Sertraline 100 mg od	Macrogol as required

Social History

Elizabeth lives alone with support from her daughters. She has no formal package of care. She has a walking stick but doesn't often use it. There are stairs in her house with a single banister rail. The only bathroom and toilet in the property is upstairs.

Examination

During examination, Elizabeth said she saw insects in the room and was picking at the bed clothes.

Chest clear, no oedema, abdomen soft and non-tender. No shortening or rotation of the right leg. Able to rotate both hips without pain, no greater trochanter tenderness, able to straight leg raise. Power and sensation grossly intact in all four limbs. Difficult to get her to relax to reliably assess limb tone.

4AT 11/12

Six-Item Screener 2/6

BP 153/78 mmHg, pulse 61 bpm, oxygen saturation 94% on air, temperature 36.8°C, glucose 5.6 mmol/L

Physiotherapy assessment: transferring from bed to chair with two-wheeled walking frame and the assistance of two people currently. Leaning back, very short shuffling steps.

Investigations

Biochemistry	Value	Reference range	Haematology	Value	Reference range
Sodium	142	133–146 mmol/L	Haemoglobin	115	115–165 g/L
Potassium	3.9	3.5–5.3 mmol/L	MCV	83	82–100 fL
Urea	5.4	2.5–7.8 mmol/L	White cell count	8.6	4–11 10^9/L
Creatinine	74	49–90 umol/L	Platelets	259	140–400 10^9/L
C-reactive protein	1	< 5 mg/L			
Adjusted calcium	2.44	2.2–2.6 mmol/L	Creatine kinase	301	25–200 U/L
TSH	2.1	0.4–4.0 mIU/L			

Liver blood tests normal

Pelvic X-ray—no fracture

What is the cause of Elizabeth's gait disturbance?
What is the cause of her hallucinations?
Should she be commenced on levodopa?
Should she be given an atypical antipsychotic, such as quetiapine?
What are the considerations for discharge planning?

Gait Disorders

A normal gait pattern requires the coordinated action of many body systems. These include the brain, peripheral nerves, muscles, joints, and balance mechanisms. Gait abnormalities often have multifactorial causation in older people. Having impaired gait and balance

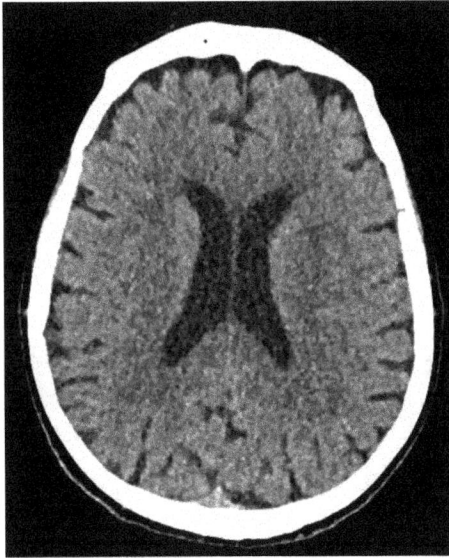

Figure 20.1 CT head showing patchy small vessel ischaemic changes.

increases the risk of falls. It may be possible to intervene to improve stability and provide appropriate mobility aids. People with cognitive impairment are at higher risk of falling. For example, they may move too fast for their level of disability or forget to use their mobility aid.

A basic gait assessment involves observing the patient standing up from sitting, walking a short distance, turning round, returning to their chair, and sitting down. If a gait abnormality is subtle, then a more difficult task, such as heel-to-toe walking, can be attempted. Table 20.1 lists aspects of gait for evaluation.

People tend to adopt a protective gait strategy in response to worrying about falling over. You can visualise what this looks like by imagining trying to walk carefully across an icy surface. Several important abnormal gait patterns are recognised and are outlined in Table 20.2. Of course, older people tend to have more than one thing wrong with them, so the picture may be mixed. 'Higher level gait disorder' is a term used for gait patterns primarily caused by brain lesions 'above' the spinal cord, cerebellum, and basal ganglia. Such a pattern can be caused by a range of neurodegenerative and vascular lesions. Higher level gait disorders include a range of appearances and can look like the gait of people with Parkinson's disease. Parkinsonism is defined as having two or more of bradykinesia, gait disturbance, rigidity, and tremor. It is very common in older people with frailty [also see Case 14].

Paratonia is a term for the clinical appearance of increased limb tone that is caused by cognitive impairment. In this scenario, the affected person tries to assist or resist passive limb movement when asked to relax. It is important to consider this when assessing tone for people with cognitive impairment.

Table 20.1 Things to Look for When Assessing Gait

Aspect	Comment
Feet	Step width—broad or narrow? (feet should be below hips) Step length High stepping (foot hanging down, knee must bend and rise more to compensate)
Body	Upright, leaning forwards, leaning backwards? Sway when walking Asymmetry
Arms	Loss of arm swing Tremor of hands
Standing up/sitting down	Need to use arms? Controlled sitting or drops into chair?
Turning around	Single smooth movement or multiple small steps? Unsteady?
Other features	Speed (< 0.8 m/s suggests abnormality) Path deviation? Unsteady? Use of aid? Freezing (i.e. failed gait initiation) Can they do tandem gait (i.e. heel-to-toe walking)?

Table 20.2 Abnormal Gait Patterns Seen in Older People

Gait pattern	Description
Hemiplegic	On the affected side: arm bent, clenched fist, straight leg, circumduction Usually caused by cerebrovascular disease
Ataxic	Broad-based, irregular pattern, unsteady appearance Can be caused by cerebellar lesions (with associated signs) or sensory disturbance (peripheral neuropathy/proprioceptive loss)
High stepping	Foot drop (unilateral/bilateral)—peripheral nerve problem See a difference in knee height from the front
Myopathic	'Waddling', difficulty standing from sitting, resultant body turning and/or swaying (hips move up and down) to compensate for proximal weakness by using upper body muscles

Gait pattern	Description
Antalgic	Due to pain, avoid prolonged weight bearing through affected limb (e.g. limp), reduced range of movement at affected joint
Higher level gait disorder (including parkinsonism)	Can be upright/stooped/hyperextended Can have freezing, feet 'stuck to the ground', shuffling Cautious gait—broad-based, slow, reduced arm swing, stooped posture, 'walking on ice', associated with fear of falling Stiffness/paratonia Often associated with cognitive impairment
Parkinsonian (i.e. Parkinson's disease)	Festination (rapid small steps to try and keep feet below forward leaning upper body), small steps, bent forwards, loss of arm swing (bradykinesia, rigidity, resting tremor, typically unilateral onset), multiple small steps when turning, freezing (gait initiation failure) Basal ganglia primarily affected—advanced disease associated with dementia

Causes of Hallucinations

Hallucinations can be related to any sensory modality but are most often visual or auditory. They commonly accompany the hyperactive subtype of delirium. They can also be caused by dementia and are frequently associated with dementia with Lewy bodies (DLB) but can occur in other forms. Sometimes they accompany severe mood disorders, which is called psychotic depression. Although associated with schizophrenia, this condition is very unlikely to present after the age of 60. Charles-Bonnet syndrome occurs when hallucinations are due to visual impairment rather than any cognitive disorder. Affected people have a disease that leads to poor vision, such as macular degeneration, but otherwise score well on cognitive tests. Medications with pro-dopaminergic effects, such as those used to treat Parkinson's disease (PD), can precipitate hallucinations. Of course, in older people with frailty, the most likely cause is a mix of several problems.

Elizabeth has previously been given a diagnostic label of 'organic hallucinosis'. In psychiatric terminology, an 'organic' disease is one in which there are measurable biological changes in body tissues that lead to symptoms, e.g. dementia. A 'non-organic', or functional, disease is one in which there are symptoms but with no measurable changes in tissues, e.g. depression. Her acute decline and initial assessment findings suggest she now also has super-imposed delirium. It is likely that there is a mixed 'acute on chronic' causation of her symptoms.

Levodopa

Levodopa is then most effective treatment for PD. It is given with a dopamine-decarboxylase inhibitor to prevent adverse effects (e.g. co-careldopa). Levodopa can cross the blood-brain barrier, whereas dopamine and decarboxylase inhibitors can't. Once within the brain, levodopa is converted to dopamine. This results in significant motor symptom improvement for people with PD. It is much less likely to have a beneficial effect on non-motor features or in other forms of parkinsonism but is sometimes tried for people with DLB. It does not have any disease-modifying effect and can cause adverse effects, including hallucinations, cognitive impairment, and OH. These are the likely reasons why Elizabeth was not felt to be suitable for a trial of this type of medication when she attended the PD clinic. During an acute episode of delirium, it doesn't feel like good time to revisit this. Should her condition change in the future, and motor symptoms suggesting PD predominate, it would be possible to reconsider a trial of medication. However, it is likely that a mix of neurodegenerative and cerebrovascular pathologies have contributed to Elizabeth's presentation.

Quetiapine

Antipsychotic medications can reduce hallucinations. Most of these medications have strong anti-dopamine effects and are contraindicated for people with PD. Some newer antipsychotics, such as quetiapine, have fewer anti-dopamine effects and probably interact with a different combination of neuroreceptor subtypes. Quetiapine has a lower risk of anti-dopamine adverse effects (e.g. worsening of parkinsonism) but higher risk of anticholinergic effects (e.g. dry mouth, constipation, and cognitive impairment). All antipsychotic medications are risky for older people with frailty, e.g. falls and aspiration pneumonia. According to the NICE guideline for Parkinson's disease, quetiapine can be considered for hallucinations for people with PD only when there is no associated cognitive impairment.[1] Additionally, clinical trial data do not support its efficacy for people with PD.[2] For all these reasons, quetiapine is very unlikely to have a net beneficial effect for Elizabeth.

What about Elizabeth?

Discharge planning for Elizabeth will be influenced by her recovery from the current illness. Her clinical presentation suggests a component of delirium, but she also has some longer-standing impairments. No obvious precipitant for delirium has been detected in her initial assessment, but triggers such as constipation and urinary retention are still possible (i.e. 'U PINCH ME' see Case 2). Her physical function is also a long way from where it was two weeks ago, e.g. mobilising independently before to now needing the assistance of two people. She requires some form of rehabilitation, which will need to be adapted to suit her degree of cognitive impairment. She may have some residual functional decline after this admission, but it is too early to know. We also need to wait until her cognitive function has been optimised to be able to assess whether she has the mental capacity to decide about her future place of residence [see Case 6].

Once we have a reasonable idea of her future needs, we can consider the barriers to going home. A clear limitation of her current property is the upstairs toilet and bathroom. Although it is possible to live upstairs in a property like this, with support, or downstairs with a commode, neither is ideal. Someone with cognitive impairment may forget their limitations and attempt to use the stairs when they are alone. Putting in a stairlift is sometimes an option.

In Elizabeth's case, a narrow staircase and lack of a landing between the top of the stairs and the bedroom door would make fitting a stairlift difficult.

Elizabeth has been reliant on support from her daughters. They have expressed concerns about her going home, and there has been recent decline. Once functionally optimised, a planning meeting may be required to ensure Elizabeth's needs are met without creating carer stress. Elizabeth and her daughters would be invited to attend along with multidisciplinary team members. Moving to a care home would be possible. If available, a property without stairs, such as sheltered accommodation, could be an appropriate yet less restrictive option. She would probably also require a formal care package to supplement the support provided by her family. Arranging all of this could take time. Sometimes, a short-term care home placement is used as an interim measure.

Delirium is likely to have contributed to Elizabeth's fall. It is also worth considering other risk factors. The description of tripping over her slipper suggests a review of her footwear is appropriate. Well-fitted, flat-soled shoes that enclose the heel are best. Depending on her discharge destination, an occupational therapist home visit to detect fall hazards could be helpful. It is possible that Elizabeth also has an element of OH. This can be assessed by measuring her lying and standing blood pressure. The sertraline and bisoprolol she is prescribed could exacerbate this and may require consideration of dose reduction, possibly leading to deprescribing.

Key Points

- Gait examination is an important aspect of geriatric assessment and can lead to useful information to help improve mobility and reduce the risk of falling.
- Dementia, delirium, visual impairment, and medication adverse effects are important things to consider when older people present with hallucinations.
- Antipsychotic medications pose a high risk of harm for older people with frailty.

Further Reading

1. National Institute for Health and Care Excellence. *Parkinson's Disease in Adults.* NICE Guideline 17. 2017. www.nice.org.uk/guidance/ng71

2. Chen JJ, Hua H, Massihi L, et al. Systematic literature review of quetiapine for the treatment of psychosis in patients with parkinsonism. *J Neuropsychiatry Clin Neurosci* 2019;31:188–95. https://doi.org/10.1176/appi.neuropsych.18080180

Case 21

Valerie

Valerie is an 87-year-old woman who was admitted following a fall at her sheltered accommodation. She had recently moved to this property, and this was the second fall in the last week. She fell overnight and was stuck on the floor for several hours, unable to summon help. Although she is significantly cognitively impaired, she was able to describe lower back pain to her carer when they found her. Valerie couldn't recall events leading up to the fall but appeared comfortable when she was assessed in the emergency department in the presence of her son and daughter.

Past Medical History

Alzheimer's dementia
Total abdominal hysterectomy and bilateral salpingo-oophorectomy 20 years ago

Medication

Donepezil 10 mg n

Social History

Valerie lives in a ground floor sheltered accommodation flat and is normally independently mobile without the use of any aids. She has a carer visit in the morning to support with medication-taking, washing, and dressing.

Examination

Valerie was awake and alert, although disoriented. She looked thin and tired, but her skin was intact. It was difficult to examine her, as she was slightly combative and didn't want to engage very much. Her daughter felt this was quite different to her usual temperament, which was amiable and chatty.

There were no signs of head or facial injury, and her arms and legs moved freely without grimacing. She was tender over the lower lumbar spine but not over the chest wall. She was able to stand and transfer to the toilet with the assistance of one person and a two-wheeled walking frame without apparent pain. Cardio-respiratory and abdominal examinations were unremarkable.

 DOI: 10.1201/9781003582007-21

Six-Item Screener 3/6
4AT 8/12
BP 127/63 mmHg, pulse 74 bpm, oxygen saturation 95% on air, temperature 36.2°C
No deficit was detected on lying-standing BP measurement.

Investigations

Biochemistry	Value	Reference range	Haematology	Value	Reference range
Sodium	138	133–146 mmol/L	Haemoglobin	104	115–165 g/L
Potassium	3.5	3.5–5.3 mmol/L	MCV	87	82–100 fL
Urea	5.5	2.5–7.8 mmol/L	White cell count	12.1	4–11 10⁹/L
Creatinine	56	49–90 umol/L	Platelets	226	140–400 10⁹/L
C-reactive protein	25	< 5 mg/L			
Albumin	33	35–50 g/L			
Adjusted calcium	2.33	2.2–2.6 mmol/L			
Alkaline phosphatase	73	30–130 IU/L			

ECG—sinus rhythm, 76 bpm
Lumbar spine X-ray – see Figure 21.1

What are the likely impacts of vertebral fractures to Valerie?
How can her risk of future fractures be reduced?

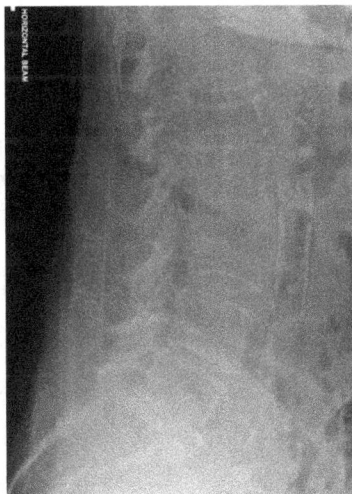

Figure 21.1 Lumbar spine X-ray showing a biconcave compression fracture of the L3 vertebral body with a reduction in height of roughly 50% centrally. There is also reduction in the height of the L1 vertebral body of approximately 40%.

Impact of Vertebral Fractures

For people who have fallen and fractured a bone, pain is a very common problem. When the bone cannot be stabilised with a cast or operative intervention, and especially if it is part of the axial skeleton (e.g. spinal or pubic rami fractures), moving around in bed, sitting, using the toilet, and attempting to stand are likely to be painful initially. Pain is often present for about six weeks—quite severe for the first couple, improving for the next two, and settling for the last. There are naturally good and bad days as increased energy and movement on one day can lead to more pain the next. The key focus is to keep mobile because taking to bed worsens pain and stiffness and results in loss of muscle and strength.[1]

Regular analgesia (that is sufficiently long acting to allow comfortable sleep), regular laxatives, and regular movement are the mainstays of treatment. For people like Valerie, with significant cognitive impairment, traditional pain scales, such as 'out of 10', are not reliable, and it is better to use validated pain scales, such as PAIN-AD or the Abbey Pain Scale, to give a more reliable assessment of whether the analgesic prescription is sufficient. If rapid progress is made with mobility, and the person is enjoying their therapy, we can be sure that pain is not holding them back, and attempts to pair back treatment can be undertaken.

Using the toilet is both difficult practically (due to assistance being required) and often painful, which can lead to constipation and urinary retention, especially when opioid analgesia is used to manage the acute severe pain. This combination puts people off their food and drink, which further exacerbates things. If the pain continues long after the usual six-week time frame, some clinicians refer to spinal surgical services for consideration of operative interventions. However, spinal vertebroplasty procedures have not been shown to be effective in reducing long-term pain when compared to sham procedures in this situation and are not routinely recommended following a Cochrane review.[2]

Thoracic vertebral fractures can lead to kyphosis (see Figure 21.2). This curvature of the spinal column can be painful. The resultant bent forward posture can affect gait and balance,

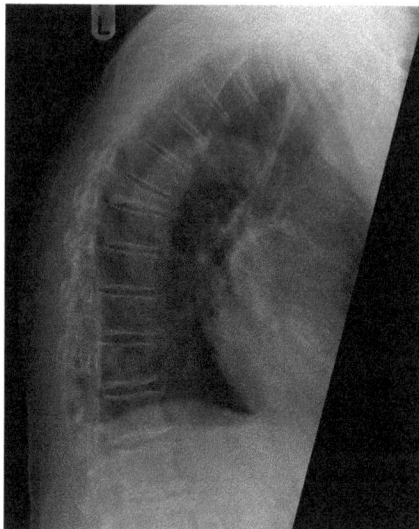

Figure 21.2 A wedge osteoporotic fracture of a mid-thoracic vertebra leads to kyphosis.

increasing the risk of falls and further fractures. Chest shape change can affect swallowing ability and, also, impair inspiration, which can potentially worsen lung conditions. The normal function of abdominal wall muscles may be altered, which can further increase the risk of constipation.

Reducing the Risk of Further Fractures

Reducing the risk of falling will reduce the risk of future fractures. CGA ensuring medical interventions such as avoidance of medications associated with increased falls risk [see Cases 4 and 8], physiotherapy interventions such as a prolonged gait and balance training programme, and home assessment to reduce trip hazards would be the foundation of an evidence-based approach to risk reduction. People with significant cognitive impairment can have limited risk awareness and can make unsafe decisions about mobilising. Personalised support measures to make it easier to access help when it is needed can be worked on with family and carers. This can include a wide range of developing technological approaches from traditional falls sensors to very sophisticated virtual carers.

Valerie's vertebral fractures occurring after a low-impact fall suggest that she has osteoporosis. In terms of osteoporosis treatments, many guidelines advocate a general approach of formal assessment of fracture risk and a threshold-based decision of whether to offer anti-resorptive treatments. The economic argument for widespread use of bone health treatments for large populations does make sense because managing the consequences of fractures is more expensive than avoiding them. Although for the individual patient, the high number needed to treat (NNT) per year to prevent a fracture may make some feel it isn't worth it for them. This coupled with the challenges of taking the medications and potential adverse effects means that in practice, many people stop taking these medications even when they have decided to try.

Fracture risk assessment using online tools, such as FRAX or QFracture, can be used to estimate the ten-year risk of fracture with high-, intermediate-, and low-risk groupings being linked to treatment recommendations. The implicit assumption is that higher risk confers greater potential benefit from treatments. In robust, community-dwelling, ambulant people, this is likely to be accurate. It is important to recognise, however, that for hospitalised older people with frailty, this may not be true for several reasons. Firstly, they often have a much shorter life expectancy than this ten-year time window. People aged over 85 in UK hospitals were found to have just under 50% mortality at one year [see Case 10], and some fractures have high associated mortality rates, e.g. following hip fracture around 30% of people aged over 80 will die in the next year.[3] In clinical trials of preventative treatments, people likely to die within a year are typically excluded. Treatments to reduce fracture risk are given for many years. People with a short life expectancy, therefore, are unlikely to complete the planned treatment before they die from any cause. There might not be time for any potential benefit to occur. These treatments are, therefore, likely to have lower efficacy. At the same time, the increased vulnerability of people with frailty raises the risk of adverse effects. Together, this affects the overall balance of risks and benefits.[4]

Vitamin D supplementation alone does not reduce fracture risk, but calcium and vitamin D combined has been shown to reduce fracture risk in meta-analyses.[5] However, most included studies are at high risk of bias. If genuine, the size of benefit is likely to be small. When anti-resorptive treatments (see later) are offered, co-prescription of vitamin D/calcium is commonplace because this was included in the design of many clinical trials.

Bisphosphonates have been common treatments to reduce fracture risk for decades. Much of the research literature focuses on reduction of vertebral fractures (morphometric, meaning seen on radiographs but without symptoms; and clinical, meaning symptomatic and confirmed on radiographs). The bisphosphonates commonly used in the UK are oral alendronate and risedronate and intravenous zoledronate. Clinical trials suggest they have similar efficacy. When communicating treatment benefits, relative risk reduction (RRR) is often used instead of absolute risk reduction (ARR). Bisphosphonates for clinical vertebral fracture have RRR 61% and ARR 1.8%.[6] This translates to a NNT of 56 people taking medication for three years to prevent one event. The equivalent numbers for hip fracture are RRR 36%, ARR 0.6%, and NNT for three years 167. This means that over 98% of people receiving treatment will not avoid these events over this period. These data will not convince everyone that medications align with their own goals. Newer medicines, such as denosumab, teriparatide, and romosozumab, have been recommended for various specific situations.[7] But the evidence for fracture risk reduction is less robust than for bisphosphonates, and each has potential adverse effects.

What about Valerie?

Valerie has moderate frailty (CFS 6). With appropriate care and rehabilitation, the hope is that she will return to her prior level of function and be able to return home, but this is not certain. She may need additional support in the short or long term. Advance care planning, probably with input from her son and daughter, is appropriate. At the time of admission, she had signs of delirium, possibly precipitated by the fall and pain from the vertebral fractures. Valerie's cognitive recovery may be prolonged, and the effects of delirium may not fully resolve.

Prior to admission, she was only prescribed one medication. Donepezil is usually recommended to be given at night. The rationale being that some people get dizziness after taking the medication and so taking at night could reduce the risk of symptoms while lying down in bed. However, this is a soft indication with unclear benefits. The timing of Valerie's donepezil was switched to the morning to enable her carer to supervise medication-taking. Ensuring that she can take the medication more consistently was judged to be most important for her.

Key Points

- Periods of immobility promote muscle loss that can have a major functional impact on people with pre-existing sarcopenia.
- Vertebral fractures can be painful, impair function, and lead to kyphosis, which may also affect walking, swallowing, breathing, and defaecating.
- Reducing the risk of falls is an important way to reduce the risk of fractures.
- Bisphosphonates reduce the risk of fracture for people with osteoporosis, but around 56 people need to take treatment for three years to prevent a clinical vertebral fracture and around 167 to prevent a hip fracture.

Further Reading

1. Rommersbach N, Wirth R, Lueg G, et al. The impact of disease-related immobilization on thigh muscle mass and strength in older hospitalized patients. *BMC Geriatr* 2020;20:500. https://doi.org/10.1186/s12877-020-01873-5

2. Buchbinder R, Johnston RV, Rischin KJ, et al. Percutaneous vertebroplasty for osteoporotic vertebral compression fracture. *Cochrane Database Syst Rev* 2018;Issue 11. Art. No.: CD006349. https://doi.org/10.1002/14651858.CD006349.pub4

3. Baji P, Patel R, Judge A, et al. Organisational factors associated with hospital costs and patient mortality in the 365 days following hip fracture in England and Wales (REDUCE): a record-linkage cohort study. *Lancet Healthy Longev* 2023;4:e386–98. https://doi.org/10.1016/S2666-7568(23)00086-7

4. Woodford HJ, Fisher J. New horizons in deprescribing for older people. *Age Ageing* 2019;48:768–75. https://doi.org/10.1093/ageing/afz109

5. Yao P, Bennett D, Mafham M, et al. Vitamin D and calcium for the prevention of fracture: a systematic review and meta-analysis. *JAMA Network Open* 2019;2:e1917789. https://doi.org/10.1001/jamanetworkopen.2019.17789

6. Goodman CW. Reconsidering the benefits of osteoporosis treatment: the case of bisphosphonates. *Am J Med* 2024;137:476–8. https://doi.org/10.1016/j.amjmed.2024.02.012

7. Qaseem A, Hicks LA, Etxeandia-Ikobaltzeta I, et al. Pharmacologic treatment of primary osteoporosis or low bone mass to prevent fractures in adults: a living clinical guideline from the American College of Physicians. *Ann Intern Med* 2023;176:224–38. https://doi.org/10.7326/M22-1034

Case 22

Elsa

Elsa is a 72-year-old former factory worker who was admitted to hospital with shortness of breath. She felt lethargic over the last week. Over the last two days, she had become breathless and developed a cough productive of clear sputum. Her oral intake had declined. She started taking her rescue pack of doxycycline and prednisolone the day prior to attending hospital, but her condition has worsened. She did not have any chest pain. She hadn't been in hospital with an exacerbation of chronic obstructive pulmonary disease (COPD) for more than a year.

Past Medical History

Acute non-ST segment elevation myocardial infarction nine years ago
COPD diagnosed 12 years ago
Mixed anxiety and depressive disorder
Mixed dementia—vascular and Alzheimer's

Medication

Aspirin 75 mg od	Beclometasone with formoterol and
Bisoprolol 5 mg od	glycopyrronium multi-dose inhaler
Carbocisteine 750 mg tds	(MDI) 87/5/9 mcg twice bd
Lansoprazole 15 mg od	Glycerol trinitrate sublingual as required
Salbutamol MDI as required	Memantine 20 mg od
	Sertraline 150 mg od

Social History

Elsa lives in a two-bedroom house. She is a current smoker. She lives with her partner, Jeremy, who is also her main carer, and he also smokes. She has poor mobility and rarely leaves the house. She struggles to get up and down the stairs. They have a pet parrot called Matilda.

Examination

Very low body mass and muscle. Chest has generalised expiratory wheeze. Heart sounds normal, no oedema. Abdomen soft and non-tender.

 DOI: 10.1201/9781003582007-22

Six-Item Screener 1/6

4AT 3/12

BP 120/64 mmHg, pulse 84 regular, oxygen saturation 93% on 40% oxygen via a mask, respiratory rate 26/min, temperature 35.6°C, weight 39.3 kg

Investigations

Biochemistry	Value	Reference range	Haematology	Value	Reference range
Sodium	142	133–146 mmol/L	Haemoglobin	126	115–165 g/L
Potassium	4.5	3.5–5.3 mmol/L	MCV	84	82–100 fL
Urea	7.4	2.5–7.8 mmol/L	White cell count	11.7	4–11 10^9/L
Creatinine	78	49–90 umol/L	Neutrophils	10.5	2.7.5 10^9/L
C-reactive protein	110	< 5 mg/L	Eosinophils	0.01	0–0.4 10^9/L
			Platelets	223	140–400 10^9/L

Arterial blood gas on 40% oxygen via a mask—pH 7.34, pCO_2 8.1, pO_2 9.7, oxygen saturation 95%, base excess 7.1, bicarbonate 32.9

Viral swab—negative for COVID/influenza

Echocardiogram two years ago: normal left ventricular size and function, mild aortic stenosis, and tricuspid regurgitation

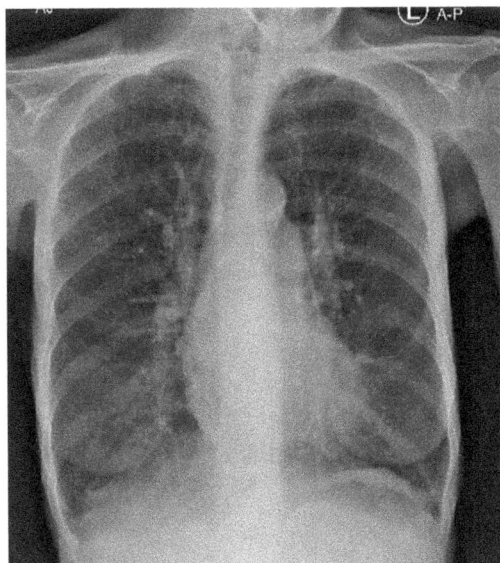

Figure 22.1 Chest X-ray showing hyperexpanded lungs.

141

Progress

Elsa was diagnosed with an acute exacerbation of COPD, possibly with an underlying bacterial chest infection (not seen on chest X-ray). She was commenced on oral steroids, nebulisers, and an intravenous broad-spectrum antibiotic. Over the next few days, her condition improved, her antibiotics were switched to oral, and her oxygen requirement reduced. Elsa is keen to get home as soon as possible. She is now receiving 1L/min of oxygen via nasal prongs. When her oxygen is removed, her saturation is measured 85 to 86% on air. She is still able to talk in full sentences.

Irene, one of Elsa's sisters, visited her in hospital and raised multiple concerns about safety at home to members of the ward team. She doesn't think that Elsa's partner, Jeremy, is assisting her with bathing properly, and Elsa is often unclean. She thinks that the house is dirty, and Elsa sits every day next to a dirty parrot cage, which has droppings all around it. She doesn't think that Elsa is eating well. She thinks that Jeremy is an alcoholic. She thinks that Jeremy's daughter from a previous marriage, Shirely, and her daughter, Michelle, are going round and taking money from Elsa without reason. She thinks that Jeremy is cutting Elsa off from Irene and her children, and they are all very concerned. She would like Shirley and Michelle to be stopped from seeing Elsa while she is in hospital.

Should Elsa be prescribed home oxygen?
How can her long-term treatment for COPD be optimised?
What are the considerations for discharge?

Home Oxygen for People with COPD

In England and Wales, NICE guidance recommends considering long-term oxygen therapy (LTOT) for nonsmokers with COPD who, on arterial blood gas testing on air, meet one of these criteria:[1]

- partial pressure of oxygen (pO_2) < 7.3 kPa
  or
- pO_2 7.3 to 7.9 kPa plus at least one of the following:
  - secondary polycythaemia
  - peripheral oedema
  - pulmonary hypertension

For people who currently smoke, smoking cessation advice +/– treatment (e.g. nicotine replacement therapy) should be offered. Home oxygen is not recommended for people who continue to smoke despite these steps. LTOT is also not recommended for isolated nocturnal hypoxaemia caused by COPD.

For delivery of LTOT, an oxygen concentrator is provided for the patient's home, along with the required tubing. LTOT assessments should consider the risk of tripping over this equipment and the risk of burns/fires (especially if living with another person who smokes). For maximum benefit, supplemental oxygen should be used for at least 15 hours per day. Ambulatory oxygen therapy can also be provided through small lightweight cylinders. This is suitable for people with COPD who desaturate with exercise, have the motivation to use oxygen, and have improved exercise capacity with oxygen use. This can provide oxygen for people when going out of their home. Specialists in the use of oxygen should be involved in the assessment of need and prescription, including optimal oxygen flow rate.

COPD Management

A combination inhaler containing a long-acting muscarinic antagonist (LAMA) and a long-acting beta 2 agonist (LABA) is standard therapy for people with COPD.[1] The addition of an inhaled steroid may be considered for people with features that suggest an element of asthma, persistent symptoms despite optimised therapy, or multiple/severe exacerbations. Having a raised serum eosinophil count also suggests a possible benefit from steroids.[2] If there is no benefit after a three-month trial, withdrawal of the steroid component can be considered. Inhaled steroids are unlikely to have the systemic adverse effects of oral steroids but do increase the risk of developing pneumonia and oropharyngeal candidiasis. Older people and current smokers are at greater risk of pneumonia.[2]

Elsa is currently prescribed a multi-dose inhaler (MDI) containing a triple combination of a LAMA, LABA, and steroid. Elsa's frailty makes her vulnerable to developing pneumonia. It would be worth establishing if she feels the steroid component has been beneficial. A trial with an inhaler containing just a LAMA and LABA would be possible.

MDI incorporate a pressurised cylinder. They have the advantage that only a low inspiratory force is required to get the drug to the small airways where they have a beneficial effect but the disadvantage of requiring coordination of the actuation with inspiration. Many people with frailty or cognitive impairment find this challenging.[2] Conversely, dry powder inhalers (DPI) have the advantage of not requiring coordination of actuation with inspiration but the disadvantage that a high inspiratory force is required to get the drug to the small airways. Assessing inhaler technique is important to choose an effective device for your patient. Using a spacer device with an MDI (not suitable for use with DPI) eliminates the need for coordination with inspiration but does add a degree of inconvenience. This simple adaptation might be helpful for Elsa.

Elsa is prescribed carbocisteine as a mucolytic, which could reduce the risk of exacerbations of COPD.[3] Continuation of this type of medication is only recommended if it results in symptomatic improvement, such as reduced cough and sputum production.[1] A potential adverse effect is increased risk of gastrointestinal bleeding. Elsa also takes aspirin and sertraline that increase this risk. Carbocysteine must be taken three times a day and contributes to medication burden. It should be established if she feels this medication is beneficial to her and a trial of withdrawal could be considered. Given that she also has a diagnosis of dementia, a trial of reduction in the dose of sertraline could be discussed [see Case 11]. Elsa's exposure to oral steroids during COPD exacerbations has increased her risk of developing osteoporosis. Consideration should be given to prescribing medications to reduce the risk of future fracture [see Case 21].

It is important that Elsa considers quitting smoking to prevent future COPD exacerbations and lung function deterioration. During her time in hospital, she was prescribed nicotine replacement therapy to reduce the risk of withdrawal symptoms, including the risk of delirium.

What about Elsa?

Elsa has stated that she is keen to return to her home. She has a diagnosis of dementia, so we need to consider if she has capacity to make this decision [see Case 6]. If not, we still need to consider her wishes and look for the least restrictive option. People have the right to make what we might consider an unwise decision. Her sister, Irene, has raised concerns, and these need to be investigated. A safeguarding referral is made due to the risk of neglect from an allegedly alcoholic partner, who is her carer, and possible financial abuse from her stepdaughter and step-granddaughter. The police may need to be involved if a crime, i.e. theft, has taken place.

Irene alleges that Jeremy has excessive alcohol intake and drinks from the early evening until the early hours of the morning. Elsa is awake during this time. He then sleeps until the afternoon and can't care for Elsa. He receives carers allowance for Elsa. Jeremy is contacted to give his side of the story. He admits that he found it stressful being the carer for Elsa and that his drinking has increased over the last few years. It is important to recognise that this is a very difficult role for him to have taken on. He has his own health issues and competing pressures from the other side of his family. Elsa has previously stated she does not want Shirley and Michelle to visit; however, Jeremy will let them in the house, where they consume alcohol together. Apparently, the police are aware and are called out to Elsa's house on a weekly basis. Elsa agreed she does not want Shirley and Michelle visiting on the ward, but she is happy for Jeremy to visit.

Irene has previously discussed with Elsa about living with her. She has the facilities for Elsa to move in with her and would like this to happen for Elsa's safety. Elsa is in agreement that this could be an option, and she would be happy to give it a try. If Elsa is living with her sister, who doesn't smoke, and was able to cease smoking herself, then LTOT could be reconsidered. She has already been receiving nicotine replacement therapy while in hospital. Clearly, this is a very complex situation. To try and find the best solution, a care planning meeting was arranged on the ward. Along with Elsa and members of the ward multi-disciplinary team, Jeremy and Irene were invited.

Key Points

- Assessing inhaler technique is important to be able to choose an effective device for your patient.
- Home oxygen therapy can be beneficial for selected people with COPD but has potential risks.
- Discharge planning can be complex.

Further Reading

1. National Institute for Health and Care Excellence. *Chronic Obstructive Pulmonary Disease in Over 16s: Diagnosis and Management*. Guideline 115. 2018. www.nice.org.uk/guidance/ng115

2. *Global Initiative for Chronic Obstructive Lung Disease Report 2023*. goldcopd.org/2023-gold-report-2/

3. Zheng J, Kang J, Huang S, et al. Effect of carbocisteine on acute exacerbation of chronic obstructive pulmonary disease (PEACE Study): a randomised placebo-controlled study. *Lancet* 2008;371:2013–8. https://doi.org/10.1016/S0140–6736(08)60869–7

Edward

Edward is an 82-year-old former accountant. He has complained of pain in his right knee for the last two or three days. He has not had a recent fall or any other form of trauma to his knee. There has been no prior knee surgery. Edward had a stroke three years ago, and this has left him with some residual right-sided weakness and expressive dysphasia. He can usually communicate his needs and opinions, but it takes him more time. He has noticed that his right knee looks more swollen than usual and feels hot to touch. He is now struggling to bend this knee or weight-bear on the joint. He thinks his urine output has reduced, the urine looks darker, and he has had some hesitancy when passing urine over the past few days. He has noted a recent mild cough but no sputum production, haemoptysis, or chest pain. His partner, Graham, has come with him to hospital. Graham thinks that Edward is more confused than usual. His temperature was recorded as 38.0°C by the ambulance crew who brought him to hospital.

Past Medical History

Epilepsy
Type 2 diabetes
Stroke—residual right-sided sided weakness and dysphasia
Anxiety

Medication

Atorvastatin 80 mg od	Clopidogrel 75 mg od
Codeine 15 mg as required	Finasteride 5 mg od
Lamotrigine 50 mg bd	Lansoprazole 30 mg od
Lisinopril 10 mg od	Metformin MR 1 g bd
Tamsulosin MR 400 mcg od	

Social History

Edward lives with his partner, Graham, who has become his main carer since the stroke. Graham had a hernia operation a few weeks ago and has since found being a carer more difficult. There is no additional care package. They live in a ground floor flat. Edward normally mobilises with a two-wheeled walker independently. He requires assistance with getting washed and dressed.

Examination

Normal alertness. Heart sounds normal. Chest clear. Abdomen soft and non-tender. No peripheral oedema. Left knee fine. Right knee warm to touch, no redness, swollen around joint compared to left, unable to tolerate passive flexion of the knee.

Six-Item Screener 4/6

4AT 5/12

BP 154/66 mmHg, pulse 95 bpm regular, oxygen saturation 94% on air, temperature 37.5°C, glucose 12.9 mmol/L

Investigations

Biochemistry	Value	Reference range	Haematology	Value	Reference range
Sodium	132	133–146 mmol/L	Haemoglobin	123	130–180 g/L
Potassium	4.4	3.5–5.3 mmol/L	MCV	89	82–100 fL
Urea	9.4	2.5–7.8 mmol/L	White cell count	14.1	4–11 10^9/L
Creatinine	80	64–104 umol/L	Neutrophils	9.9	2–7.5 10^9/L
C-reactive protein	86	< 5 mg/L	Platelets	122	140–400 10^9/L
Uric acid	412	200–430 umol/L			

Liver blood tests and calcium normal
Hb$_{A1C}$ 55 mmol/mol three months ago
Viral swab for influenza/COVID negative

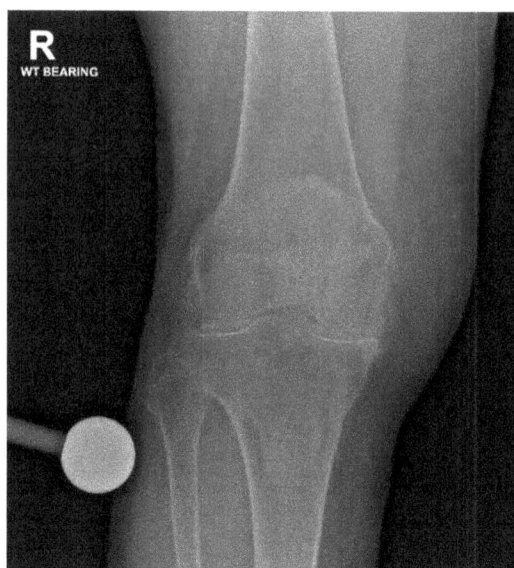

Figure 23.1 X-ray of right knee showing chondrocalcinosis.

What causes of an acute inflamed knee need to be considered?
What are the discharge considerations for Edward?

Acute Joint Inflammation

There are several possible causes of an acutely inflamed joint in an older person. The most likely are discussed in the following sections.

Osteoarthritis

Osteoarthritis (OA) is the most common joint disorder, and it becomes more common with advancing age. Pathologic changes include loss of cartilage, osteophyte formation, bone sclerosis, and cyst formation around the joint margins. These changes can be seen on X-ray images. The usual presentation is with painful and stiff joints. Sometimes joints can become swollen or tender. There may be associated crepitation when moving the joint. Analgesia, physiotherapy, increasing exercise, and optimising weight can help. Severe cases may be considered for joint replacement surgery. Acute joint flare-ups can occur with OA in the absence of trauma and could increase pain and swelling in the affected joint. For Edward, his raised temperature, serum WCC, and C-reactive protein suggest this is more than an OA flare.

Rheumatoid Arthritis

Rheumatoid arthritis (RA) is the commonest inflammatory joint disorder. It most commonly affects peripheral, smaller joints, such as metacarpophalangeal and proximal interphalangeal joints. Sometimes larger joints are affected. Morning stiffness lasting more than an hour is characteristic. In Edward's case, RA presenting as a single swollen knee would be very unusual.

Gout

Gout is caused by monosodium urate crystal deposition with a joint. It most commonly affects the hands and feet, especially the first toe. In older people, it is associated with diuretic use, obesity, impaired renal function, and myeloproliferative disease. Chronic gout can lead to the formation of tophi (accumulations of monosodium urate crystals on the fingers, toes, or elbows). Serum urate levels are not very helpful for diagnosing gout but can be used to guide treatment for the prevention of future exacerbations (e.g. prescribing an effective dose of allopurinol). Acute exacerbations can be controlled with a short oral course of prednisolone, a non-steroidal anti-inflammatory drug NSAIDs or colchicine.[1] NSAIDs have multiple potential adverse effects and are usually avoided in older people with frailty. Colchicine often causes diarrhoea. Although prednisolone has many potential adverse effects, short courses at a low dose are usually well tolerated.

Calcium Pyrophosphate Deposition Disease (CPPD, or 'Pseudogout')

CPPD is caused by calcium pyrophosphate deposition with a joint. It most commonly affects the knee, followed by the wrist. Chronic CPPD can resemble OA. X-rays may show deposition of calcium on the articular cartilage, which is called chondrocalcinosis. Acute management is the same as for gout. There is no long-term risk reduction treatment (i.e. analogous to allopurinol for gout) for pseudogout.

Septic Arthritis

Septic arthritis is difficult to distinguish clinically from a flare of inflammatory arthritis or an attack of gout or CPPD. Joint aspiration is the best way to find out. Septic arthritis is more likely to occur in people with a history of RA, prosthetic joints, diabetes, age over 80, or superimposed skin infection. The knee and shoulder joints are the most affected. Staphylococci and streptococci are the commonest causative organisms. Management requires intravenous antibiotics and urgent referral to an orthopaedic team.

What about Edward?

Edward was seen by the orthopaedic team, and an aspiration of his right knee was performed in the emergency department. Calcium pyrophosphate crystals were detected in the aspirate. No organisms were seen, and no bacterial growth was detected. This established the diagnosis as CPPD and excluded septic arthritis. He was prescribed a course of oral steroids—prednisolone 15 mg od for seven days. Although this could worsen his diabetic control, it was felt to be a better option than an NSAID or colchicine for him. His blood glucose would need to be monitored more closely during this treatment. His knee inflammation improved over the next few days and his delirium resolved. The physiotherapy team were able to get him mobile enough to go home again. Some ongoing community rehabilitation was arranged to continue in his own home until he had fully recovered.

Since the stroke, Graham has taken on the challenging additional role of being Edward's carer. He has done a great job for the past three years. Understandably, while he is recovering from his own operation, he has found things more difficult. We need to establish that Graham still feels he can support Edward. It may be helpful to provide a short-term package of care. This would give Graham more chance to recover and see if having carers would be beneficial in the future. Graham is also in his eighties and has several health problems. He is concerned he may not be able to support Edward for much longer.

Edward has moderate frailty (CFS 6). His main goal is to live with Graham in their flat for as long as possible. If he were to develop a serious health condition, then he would not want any treatment that could result in him surviving with increased functional impairment. An agreement is made to complete a 'do not resuscitate' form for him.

Key Points

- Septic arthritis needs to be considered for people presenting with an acutely inflamed joint.
- CPPD often presents as a swollen knee or wrist.

- It is important to consider the needs of current carers when planning discharge from hospital.

Further Reading

1. Billy CA, Lim RT, Ruospo M, et al. Corticosteroid or nonsteroidal antiinflammatory drugs for the treatment of acute gout: a systematic review of randomized controlled trials. *J Rheumatol* 2018;45:128–36. https://doi.org/10.3899/jrheum.170137

Janet

Janet is an 88-year-old woman who came to hospital following an unwitnessed fall at home. She was trying to get to the toilet when she fell but can't recall exactly how it occurred. Her mobility has declined recently. She struggles to walk due to pain and swelling of both legs, which is a longstanding problem. Her GP had recently prescribed codeine to help with pain control. She says the pain in her left lower leg has worsened since the fall. She is struggling to put weight through that limb now. She has not had any chest or urine symptoms. Her family members are concerned that her cognition has been deteriorating over the last few months.

Past Medical History

Cerebral amyloid angiopathy (CAA) diagnosed a year ago on brain scans done to investigate cognitive impairment
Organic hallucinosis six years ago
Anxiety
Osteoarthritis—previous left hip and right knee joint replacement surgeries
Hypertension
Vitamin B_{12} deficiency
Asthma

Medication

Atorvastatin 40 mg od	Codeine 15 mg qds
Colecalciferol 800 units od	Furosemide 20 mg od
Hydroxocobalamin 1 mg three-monthly	Ibuprofen 5% gel as required
Lisinopril 30 mg od	Loratadine 10 mg as required
Melatonin 2 mg MR n	Paracetamol 1 g qds
Propranolol 40 mg tds	Salbutamol inhaler as required
Senna 7.5 mg n	

Social History

Janet lives alone since her husband died four years ago. She uses a single stick when walking around her property, and she no longer goes out alone. There is a stairlift in her house. She has carers twice a day to assist with getting washed, dressed, and meal preparation. Her son also visits two or three times each week and does her shopping.

 DOI: 10.1201/9781003582007-24

Examination

Chest clear. Heart sounds normal. Abdomen soft and non-tender. Non-pitting lymphoedema of both legs. She reports pain with even very small movements of either leg. No obvious deformity. Scars from previous joint surgery. Unable to stand with the assistance of two people. No signs of head injury.

Six-Item Screener 0/6

4AT 3/12

BP variable 113/63 to 190/78 mmHg (couldn't stand to do lying and standing measurements), pulse regular 77 bpm, oxygen saturation 97% on air, temperature 36.1°C, weight 84.7 kg

Investigations

Biochemistry	Value	Reference range	Haematology	Value	Reference range
Sodium	147	133–146 mmol/L	Haemoglobin	122	115–165 g/L
Potassium	3.7	3.5–5.3 mmol/L	MCV	93	82–100 fL
Urea	4.0	2.5–7.8 mmol/L	White cell count	7.4	4–11 10^9/L
Creatinine	58	49–90 umol/L	Platelets	211	140–400 10^9/L
C-reactive protein	2	< 5 mg/L			
Creatine kinase	582	25–200 IU/L			

Liver blood tests and calcium normal

Janet went on to have a CT scan of her pelvis, which also didn't show a fracture.

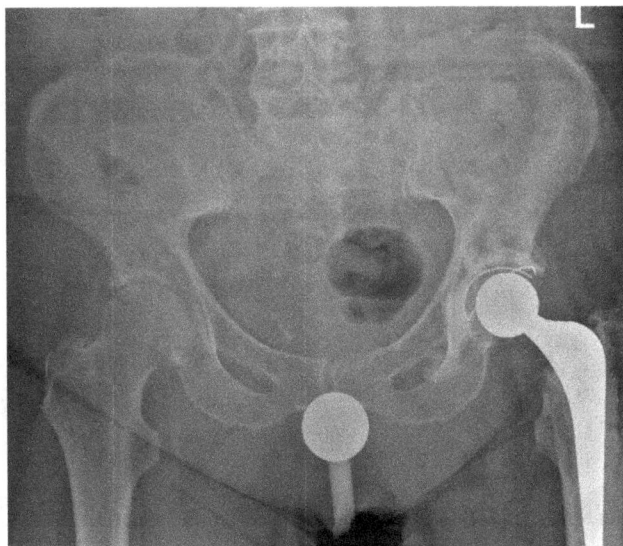

Figure 24.1 Pelvic X-ray showing old left hip surgery and some osteoarthritic changes in her right hip but no fracture.

What is cerebral amyloid angiopathy?
What is the cause of Janet's leg pain?

Cerebral Amyloid Angiopathy

CAA is the deposition of amyloid protein (amyloid-beta) in the intracerebral blood vessel walls.[1] This can damage blood vessel integrity, leading to intracranial haemorrhage (ICH) and cognitive decline. The bleeds are usually found in the cerebral cortex, whereas bleeds in subcortical regions and the cerebellum are more commonly associated with hypertension. The onset of bleeds is usually non-traumatic. It has increasing prevalence in older age and is associated with Alzheimer's dementia neuropathology, which leads to intracerebral amyloid deposition, and in autopsy studies has been found in 90% of cases. CAA is usually detected by MRI imaging using gradient echo sequences, which can detect haemosiderin deposits, whereas CT imaging can only detect acute bleeds that have occurred within the last week (see Figure 24.2). Many cases are likely to be unrecognised. Imaging studies suggest that CAA affects 20–40% of the population aged over 80 without cognitive impairment and 50–60% of those with cognitive impairment. No treatment is currently available. An important clinical consideration is its associated increased risk of ICH with anticoagulants/antiplatelets. This probably explains the doubling of bleeding risk in people with cognitive impairment [see Case 11].

Janet's Leg Pain

The longstanding nature of Janet's pain and the absence of an acute abnormality on imaging make a traumatic aetiology less likely. The cause is not immediately obvious. Like many presentations in older people, it may be a combination of several factors. She is known to

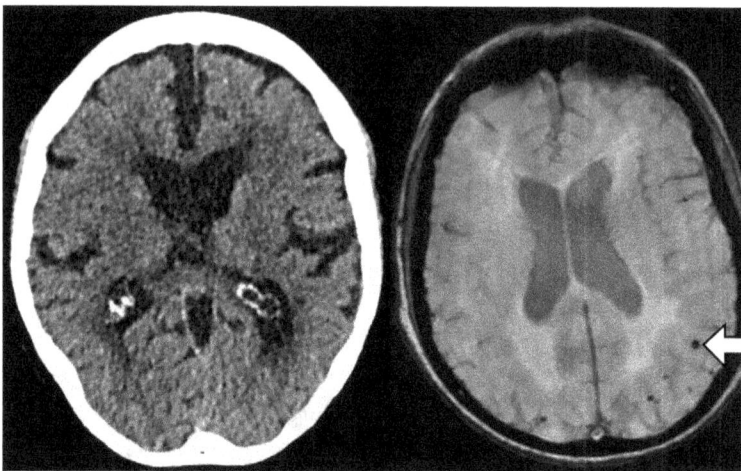

Figure 24.2 Brain imaging showing CAA. CT scan (left) shows atrophy and small vessel ischaemia only. MRI scan (right) shows small dark circles (arrow), on gradient echo sequences, representing prior intracerebral bleeds.

have osteoarthritis. She has lymphoedema of her legs, which can be painful. Furosemide is unlikely to have much impact for lymphoedema. If her circulation permits, compression bandages could be tried instead. There may be an element of anxiety, made worse by cognitive impairment and being in an unfamiliar hospital environment. The pain seemed to come on with only minimal leg movement. Sometimes statin medications can cause myalgia.[2] Her creatine kinase is a little raised, but this may be due to her recent fall. Muscle symptoms can occur without a rise in creatine kinase and are more likely to occur in older people with frailty.[3] Even mild muscle symptoms could have a major functional impact on someone with sarcopenia. Janet doesn't have a strong indication to continue taking a statin. It is worth discussing whether she would like to try a 'holiday' off this medication to see if her symptoms improve without it. The codeine that her GP prescribed doesn't seem to have helped much and could worsen cognition and increase the risk of falling. Switching to an alternative medication is an option, but all have some potential adverse effects.

What about Janet?

Janet has moderate frailty (CFS 6), and her condition has been declining. Her limited mobility and cognitive impairment make her vulnerable at home alone. We need to try and improve her leg pain and get her mobile again. Once we have seen how she progresses, we can start to consider the issues that will need to be address at the time of discharge. She has limited life expectancy, and a conversation about advance care planning should be had with Janet and her son. It would be important to discuss the value of continuing or stopping the other medicines that might increase her risk of falling (e.g. lisinopril, propranolol) in this context.

Key Points

- CAA commonly occurs in older people with cognitive impairment and increases the risk of intracerebral bleeding.
- Symptoms in older people with frailty can have multifactorial causation, and interventions may need to be multifaceted.

Further Reading

1. Cozza M, Amadori L, Boccardi V. Exploring cerebral amyloid angiopathy: insights into pathogenesis, diagnosis, and treatment. *J Neurological Sci* 2023;454:120866. https://doi.org/10.1016/j.jns.2023.120866

2. Parker BA, Capizzi JA, Grimaldi AS, et al. Effect of statins on skeletal muscle function. *Circulation* 2013;127:96–103. https://doi.org/10.1161/CIRCULATIONAHA.112.136101

3. Nguyen KA, Li L, Lu D, et al. A comprehensive review and meta-analysis of risk factors for statin-induced myopathy. *Eur J Clin Pharmacol* 2018;74:1099–109. https://doi.org/10.1007/s00228-018-2482-9

Joseph

Joseph is a 74-year-old retired builder who is seen in the out-patient clinic. A few weeks ago, he had an annual health check, and at the time, his systolic BP was greater than 200 mmHg. He had a history of hypertension and vascular disease. His doctor increased his amlodipine dose from 5 to 10 mg daily. However, the following week, his BP was even higher with systolic 220 mmHg. Ramipril was added to his other medications. Joseph was now very concerned that he might have another stroke and if something else was wrong with him to make his BP so high. A 24-hour BP monitor was requested, and he was referred to the out-patient clinic. Other than worrying about his BP, Joseph was feeling ok and had no new symptoms.

Past Medical History

Stroke ten years ago—no residual neurological deficit
Ischaemic heart disease
Type 2 diabetes
Hypertension
Mild cognitive impairment
Anxiety

Medication

Amitriptyline 20 mg n	Amlodipine 10 mg od
Atorvastatin 80 mg od	Calcium/vitamin D tablet bd
Clopidogrel 75 mg od	Gliclazide 80 mg bd
Metformin MR 1 g bd	Ramipril 5 mg od
Ranolazine MR 375 mg bd	Sitagliptin 100 mg od

Social History

Joseph lives with his wife in a house. He is independently mobile and does not need any help with activities of daily living. Over the last couple of years, he has been less active and tends to spend most of his day at home watching the television. He rarely drinks alcohol and stopped smoking after his stroke ten years ago.

DOI: 10.1201/9781003582007-25

Examination

Normal alertness. Heart sounds normal. Chest clear. No peripheral oedema. Abdomen soft and non-tender. Ophthalmoscopy did not show any significant changes.

Six-Item Screener 5/6

4AT 0/12

BP 192/76 mmHg, pulse 68 bpm, oxygen saturation 96% on air, temperature 36.8°C, weight 96.4 kg

Investigations

Biochemistry	Value	Reference range	Haematology	Value	Reference range
Sodium	139	133–146 mmol/L	Haemoglobin	136	130–180 g/L
Potassium	4.5	3.5–5.3 mmol/L	MCV	89	82–100 fL
Urea	6.2	2.5–7.8 mmol/L	White cell count	7.6	4–11 10^9/L
Creatinine	109	64–104 umol/L	Platelets	281	140–400 10^9/L
Adjusted calcium	2.24	2.2–2.6 mmol/L			
Total vitamin D	77	> 50 nmol/L	Hb$_{A1C}$	61	20–41 mmol/mol
TSH	1.7	0.3–4.5 mIU/L			

ECG—sinus rhythm 72 bpm, no ischaemic changes

24-hour BP recording (see Figure 25.1): overall average BP 133/65 mmHg, daytime average 119/63 mmHg, nighttime average 145/68 mmHg, and lowest BP 84/48 mmHg

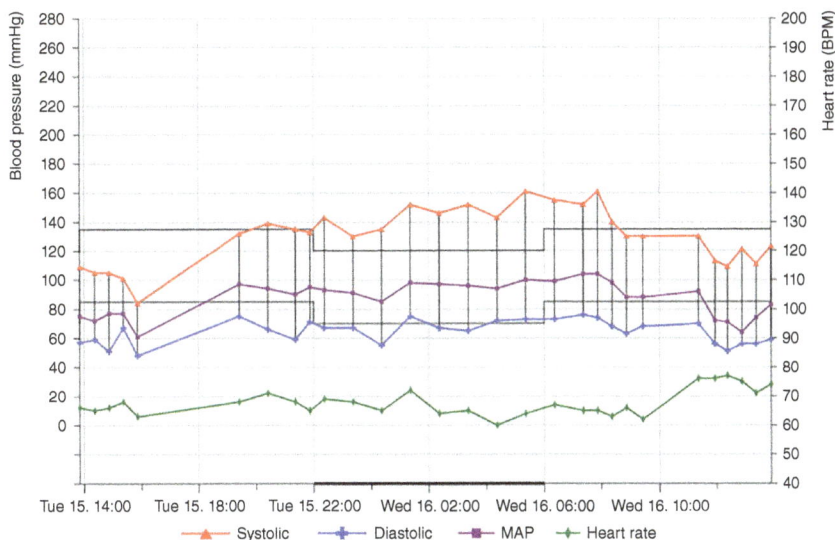

Figure 25.1 24-hour BP recording.

Why is Joseph's clinic BP higher than the 24-hour average?
Is his higher nighttime BP relevant?
Why is his BP sometimes low?
How would you optimise his BP control?

White Coat Effect

White coat hypertension is a term for finding elevated BP measurements in clinical settings while having non-elevated measurements on home or ambulatory assessments. Unfortunately, it has an old-fashioned name relating back to when only doctors in white coats measured BP. White coat effect is a common finding. It may be triggered by anxiety, including health-related anxiety, leading to increased sympathetic nervous system activity. It may not be a benign condition and has been associated with elevated risk of adverse cardiovascular outcomes in some studies.[1]

Because white coat effect is common, ambulatory BP monitoring is a useful tool to help assess BP control for people with hypertension and reduce the risk of inadvertent over-treatment potentially leading to medication-related harm. Average BP with ambulatory recording should be a little lower than clinic measurements. In England and Wales, NICE guidelines recommend a daytime target of 135/85 mmHg or lower for people aged under 80, compared to a target of below 140/90 mmHg for clinic readings.[2] For people with white coat hypertension, lifestyle advice to reduce the risk of developing cardiovascular disease (i.e. reduced salt and alcohol intake, optimise weight, healthy diet, and increased exercise) is appropriate, but there is no clear evidence that prescribing antihypertensive medications improves outcomes.

Nocturnal Hypertension

In the normal physiological state, nighttime average BP is a little lower than average daytime BP. Nocturnal hypertension is a term for having high BP overnight, which can occur when daytime BP is not elevated (called 'isolated nocturnal hypertension') and is usually only detected through ambulatory 24-hour BP monitoring.[3] Consequently, it is likely to be underdiagnosed, and an accurate prevalence is unknown. It is associated with older age, high salt intake, obesity, nocturia, obstructive sleep apnoea (OSA), diabetes, chronic kidney disease, and various cardiovascular diseases.

Several mechanisms could cause nighttime BP to rise. People with peripheral oedema could have increased reabsorption of fluid from the legs while lying flat, leading to increased venous return to the heart. People with nocturia could have a rise in sympathetic tone in response to a distended bladder. Similarly, people with OSA could have increased sympathetic activity in response to hypoxia. Taking shorter acting BP-lowering medications in the morning could lead to a relatively higher BP overnight after the medication effects have diminished. Keeping a diary of overnight activity and symptoms may help to identify potential exacerbating factors.

Although not specifically tested in clinical trials, periods of high BP at any time of the day are likely to promote organ damage, and avoiding high BP with medications probably reduces this risk. It doesn't appear to influence outcomes whatever time of day long-acting hypertensives are taken.[4] And making the timing of medicine-taking more complex could reduce adherence. Taking shorter-acting antihypertensives at bedtime has been suggested for some people with OH during the day and high BP while lying down at night, but there is no clinical trial evidence to support safety or efficacy.[5] Such a strategy could increase the risk of low BP episodes overnight, for example, if getting out of bed to go to the toilet.

Orthostatic Hypotension

Joseph's intermittent low BP could represent episodes of OH [see Case 11], which is associated with supine hypertension, possibly through changes in baroreceptor function in response to chronic BP elevation. Biological ageing leads to increased stiffness of large blood vessels and tends to increase this association. Autonomic nervous system dysfunction could also play a role. When OH is suspected, BP should be measured while sitting/lying and one minute after standing.[2] When a difference is detected, the lower BP value obtained should be used to guide treatment decisions. If a postural drop in BP is asymptomatic, then maybe no action is required. It is worth asking if the person feels light-headed on standing and if they have ever had any falls or episodes of loss of consciousness.

Optimising Jospeh's BP Control

Joseph has a combination of isolated nocturnal hypertension and episodes of low daytime BP, possibly with OH. BP control starts with non-pharmacological approaches. Joseph's weight is 96.4 kg, which gives him a body mass index of 31, indicating obesity. Optimising his weight could help to lower his BP. This could be achieved through modifying his diet and increasing exercise. He has been less active over the last two years. Reducing the salt in his diet may also help. Cutting back alcohol intake is relevant for some people, but Joseph is not a regular drinker. These steps in combination could significantly lower his BP without the risk of medication adverse effects, including OH.

We should look for other factors that could increase his nocturnal BP. OSA is commonly associated with obesity. It is caused by the collapse of upper airways during sleep, leading to apnoeic episodes and hypoxia.[6] In response, increased sympathetic nervous system activity promotes nocturnal hypertension. Periods of arousal are trigged that fragment sleep, leading to daytime sleepiness and fatigue. There may also be associated morning headaches. Joseph's wife may have noticed excessive snoring, gasping/choking noises, or apnoeic episodes during the night. A formal diagnosis is made with sleep studies that assess respiratory parameters. Weight loss and exercise can help. If severe, a continuous positive airway pressure mask worn overnight could improve symptoms and lower his nighttime BP. We should also ask about nocturia [see Case 13]. He is at risk of benign prostatic hyperplasia. Medications or a procedure to reduce the size of his prostate gland could help prevent nocturnal hypertension due to sympathetic nervous activity in response to a distended bladder. Optimising sleep hygiene may also be useful.

Recognising that medication adherence is seldom perfect, we should not assume that Joseph always takes all his medication as prescribed. The subject should be sensitively explored with him, trying to establish that prescribing is in accordance with his own goals and if there are any barriers that could be addressed. The antihypertensive medications that

Joseph is prescribed (ramipril and amlodipine) are long-acting and should provide 24-hour BP control irrespective of what time of day they are taken. He is also prescribed ranolazine, for angina, that can cause hypotension that may only affect his daytime BP. We should ask if he has had any recent angina. It would be possible to switch him to an alternative, such as a long-acting beta blocker, to see if this had less effect on his daytime BP.

What about Joseph?

Joseph is not frail but has become less active and is at risk of developing frailty (CFS 4). He is very worried about his high BP recordings and the future risk of stroke. One aspect of his management is reassurance that the 24-hour BP recording has shown that his BP is lower than the few times it has been measured in clinic settings. His known anxiety may play a role in this difference. He is prescribed amitriptyline for this symptom. Given this drug has strong anticholinergic effects, it could be contributing to his mild cognitive impairment and potentially worsen any OH symptoms. An alternative medication, such as a selective serotonin reuptake inhibitor, might be a better option for him.

Key Points

- White coat hypertension (elevated BP measurements in clinical settings while having non-elevated measurements on home or ambulatory assessments) is common.
- 24-hour BP monitoring can assess hypertension control, reduce the risk of inadvertent overtreatment, and detect nocturnal hypertension.
- Nocturnal hypertension can be caused by OSA or nocturia.
- OH is commonly associated with supine hypertension—making management more challenging.
- Non-pharmacological measures for optimising BP control should not be overlooked.

Further Reading

1. Nuredin G, Saunders A, Rajkumar C, et al. Current status of white coat hypertension: where are we? *Ther Adv Cardiovasc Dis* 2020;14:1–10. https://doi.org/10.1177/1753944720931637

2. National Institute for Health and Care Excellence. *Hypertension in Adults: Diagnosis and Management.* NG136. 2019.

3. Liu J, Li Y, Zhang X, et al. Management of nocturnal hypertension: an expert consensus document from Chinese Hypertension League. *J Clin Hypertens* 2024;26:71–83. https://doi.org/10.1111/jch.14757

4. Mackenzie IS, Rogers A, Poulter NR, et al. Cardiovascular outcomes in adults with hypertension with evening versus morning dosing of usual antihypertensives in the UK (TIME study): a prospective, randomised, open-label, blinded-endpoint clinical trial. *Lancet* 2022;400:1417–25. https://doi.org/10.1016/S0140–6736(22)01786-X

5. Jordan J, Fanciulli A, Tank J, et al. Management of supine hypertension in patients with neurogenic orthostatic hypotension: scientific statement of the American Autonomic Society, European Federation of Autonomic Societies, and the European Society of Hypertension. *J Hypertens* 2019;37:1541–6. https://doi.org/10.1097/HJH.0000000000002078

6. Gottlieb DJ, Punjabi NM. Diagnosis and management of obstructive sleep apnea: a review. *JAMA* 2020;323:1389–400. https://doi.org/10.1001/jama.2020.3514

Beatrice

Beatrice is a 67-year-old woman who presented with loss of consciousness, abdominal pain, and vomiting. Her son rang for an ambulance after she had 'blacked out' at home. This happened after a few hours of abdominal pain followed by an episode of vomiting dark-coloured liquid. She had been constipated for a few weeks prior to all this. She was clearly unwell in the emergency department, and an urgent assessment by the surgical team and a CT scan led to a diagnosis of severe constipation and stercoral perforation.

Past Medical History

Left partial anterior circulation stroke followed by intracranial haemorrhage a year ago
Post-stroke seizures
Diet-controlled type 2 diabetes
Hypertension
Constipation

Medication

Atorvastatin 20 mg od	Clopidogrel 75 mog od
Docusate 200 mg bd	Lansoprazole 30 mg od
Levetiracetam 500 mg bd	Lisinopril 10 mg od
Mirabegron 50 mg od	

Social History

Beatrice had been living with her son, in his house, since having a stroke. She was independent with self-care but has some residual expressive dysphasia. She could mobilise with a stick at home but only went out with her son. She can go up and down the stairs without difficulty.

Surgery and Early Recovery

Beatrice underwent emergency surgery, which removed the section of damaged bowel and formed a colostomy (i.e. Hartmann's procedure). She went to critical care post-operatively,

 DOI: 10.1201/9781003582007-26

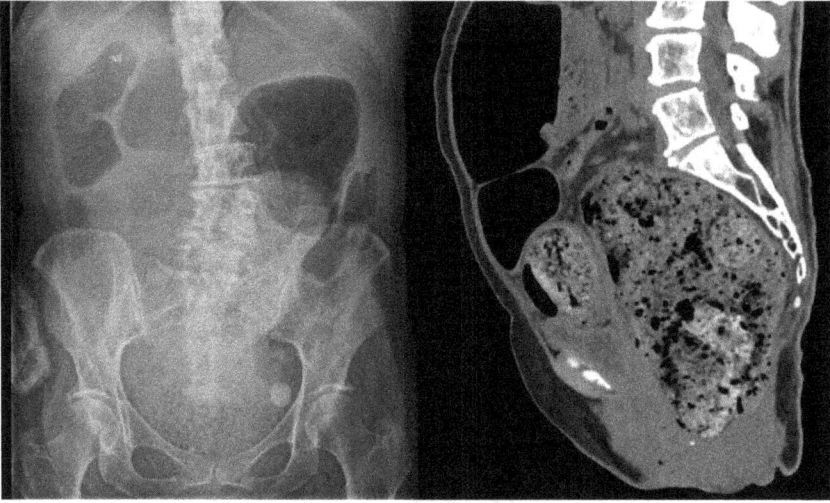

Figure 26.1 Abdominal X-ray and CT scan showing a large faecal mass in the rectum with dilated bowel above.

where she was initially shocked and septic, requiring antibiotics, vasopressors, intubation, and ventilation. She had intravenous total parenteral nutrition in the early phase of her treatment, followed by nasogastric feeding due to having an impaired swallow following her severe illness. Her BP remained relatively low even without the lisinopril, which was withheld as part of the early treatment of her septic shock. As she improved and her more invasive treatments were no longer necessary, it became clear that she was markedly delirious but fortunately did not develop other acute medical complications. Her mobility improved with therapy, and her delirium became less distressing. She continued to find it very difficult to engage with her new stoma, though. She would not look at it when the nurses changed the bag and didn't want to talk about it.

> **Could Beatrice's constipation and faecal impaction have been managed better?**
> **How would you approach her acute admission with abdominal pain?**
> **What factors affect the chance of returning to independent living following emergency surgery?**

Constipation and Faecal Impaction

Constipation is a very common symptom for older people with frailty. Many find a routine that allows them to comfortably manage their bowels over many years. Abrupt changes to mobility (e.g. having a stroke or following a fracture) can precipitate rapid change in bowel function, as can the prescription of constipating medications (e.g. opioids or anticholinergics). Management of constipation focusses on improving oral food and fluid intake and mobilisation [see Case 18]. Laxatives can help, and the choice depends on whether someone is mobile and what their oral intake is like. Bulking agents should be avoided when immobile or with reduced intake (i.e. most older people with frailty in hospital). Docusate has not been shown to be effective as a laxative and is a good candidate for deprescribing.[1] Stimulants (e.g. bisacodyl/senna) and osmotic laxatives (e.g. lactulose/macrogol) are effective and can be selected depending on oral intake.

Faecal impaction is a build-up of large hard stools. This is thought to be related to the impairment of normal physiological response to stools entering the rectum that usually triggers defaecation.

Increasing volume of stool in the rectum can have knock-on effects of urinary retention or incontinence, faecal incontinence, and rarely, ulceration of the bowel and even perforation. Treatment of faecal impaction is usually with a combination of oral laxatives and rectal suppositories or enemas. Rarely, manual evacuation is necessary to relieve the impaction. For Beatrice, there was a missed opportunity to switch to a more effective laxative regime in the lead-up to her admission in crisis.

Abdominal Pain

Like 'medical' diagnoses, older people with frailty who have 'surgical' illnesses (e.g. cholecystitis, bowel obstruction, ischaemia, or perforation) have a much poorer prognosis than non-frail people. It is also more difficult to make diagnoses for those with cognitive impairment. On top of the insult from the intra-abdominal pathology, associated reduction in oral intake leads rapidly to undernourishment and dehydration. There is a high risk of delirium, decreased mobility, and falls.

Many regional guidelines advocate review by a senior surgeon within an hour when someone presents to hospital with abdominal pain so severe that they require intravenous analgesia or associated with abnormal physiological signs (e.g. hypotension or tachycardia). This is because rapid diagnosis, decision-making, and intervention is critical in the presence of bowel obstruction or perforation with associated sepsis. Delaying surgery worsens outcomes and so international consensus recommends operating within six hours. Early review of their prescription should focus on medicines that can worsen the symptoms. These include constipating agents [see Case 18] and gastric irritants (e.g. NSAID, bisphosphonates) but also those that increase the chance of organ dysfunction (e.g. antihypertensive medications reducing renal perfusion, anticholinergic medications increasing risk of delirium).

In England, the National Emergency Laparotomy Audit is a quality improvement project that captures data on all people underdoing emergency surgery.[2] Through many iterations, it has led to recommendations about early assessment and scanning, senior surgeons and anaesthetists being present in theatre, and planned admission to critical care post-operatively when mortality risk is greater than 5%. More recent recommendations include input from specialists in geriatric medicine for older people with frailty undergoing surgery. This can help to coordinate the multidisciplinary teams involved in returning to independence after surgery. Hospitals where this recommendation is routinely implemented have lower mortality following emergency surgery. Evidence around enhanced recovery after surgery in the emergency setting is building, and international guidelines have been published to try to improve care for this group of patients.[3, 4] Specific focus on reducing anticholinergic/sedative burden in the operative period, reducing opioid use by local anaesthetic wound treatments, and avoiding unduly deep anaesthesia by using monitoring are examples of how a focus on factors that influence delirium incidence can be built into high-quality standard care.

What about Beatrice?

Beatrice was mildly frail (CFS 5) prior to her operation. She needed input from a broad multi-disciplinary team, all of whom supported her journey through severe illness back to independence. Emergency physicians, surgeons, anaesthetists, geriatricians, nurses, pharmacists, dietitians, speech and language therapists, physiotherapists, occupational therapists, and stoma nurses all brought specific technical skills and worked with Beatrice and her family to understand what was happening to her.

A major challenge for people having surgery is delirium. The necessary polypharmacy of anaesthesia coupled with the inflammatory storm of their illness and the multiple care environments make this very common (more than 60% of people in our local data). One of the big issues facing people with emergency surgery is accepting a new body image. Stomas are strange things for people to come to terms with in the elective surgical setting, and in the context of delirium and emergency surgery, they can be incomprehensible. Psychological support around validating the sense of strangeness of having been operated on, not really understanding what has happened 'inside', and the memories of fear and distress related to delirium is vital. Beatrice really struggled with coming to terms with her new stoma, and her delirium on top of the physical impairments and dysphasia from her previous stroke increased the challenge. Fortunately, her husband was both willing and able to learn how to manage it for her. As well as delirium, other factors that reduce the chance of survival to independent living after emergency surgery include high preoperative risk (based on physical and functional parameters and the acute illness features) and unplanned return to theatre. These are all frequently a concern for patients, family, and staff alike, and their presence should lead to honest conversations about realistic outcome goals as the situation develops.

Having cut down many of her medications in the very early phase of her admission, Beatrice's oral intake did improve, and whether to restart her longer-term medications was discussed. Several useful factors to consider in this circumstance include the following:

1) Prioritising early recovery—getting back to normal eating and toileting habits are positive. What medication will help or hinder this? Those causing GI symptoms are worth avoiding, for example.
2) Long-term prognostication may have changed. If someone hasn't recovered well and is significantly more dependent than prior to their operation, long-term risk reduction medications may no longer be of significant value.
3) Low blood pressure following emergency surgery can last some weeks. It is unclear why some people who previously took several antihypertensives require none following a big operation. Reintroducing them when the blood pressure is already low may increase the risk of falls and impaired organ function, so pausing them and then reviewing their need within a few weeks of return home can be sensible.

After discussion, we agreed to stay off the lisinopril and mirabegron, as her blood pressure remained low and she had suffered with urinary retention while in hospital. Beatrice was able to return home with her husband, along with some regular support for washing and dressing, and assistance with her stoma.

Key Points

- Constipation can be enormously burdensome, and appropriate lifestyle advice and effective laxatives are the mainstay of treatment.
- Delirium is a frequent complication of post-surgical care for older people.
- Emergency surgery is a significant insult for an older person with frailty, and survival requires coordinated multi-disciplinary working with a focus on recovery to independence.

Further Reading

1. Fakhiri RJ, Volpicelli FM. Things we do for no reason: prescribing docusate for constipation in hospitalized adults. *J Hospital Med* 2019;14:110–3. https://doi.org/10.12788/jhm.3124

2. www.nela.org.uk

3. Peden CJ, Aggarwal G, Aitken RJ, et al. Guidelines for perioperative care for emergency laparotomy Enhanced Recovery After Surgery (ERAS) Society recommendations: part 1—preoperative: diagnosis, rapid assessment and optimization. *World J Surgery* 2021;45:1272–90. https://doi.org/10.1007/s00268-021-05994-9

4. Scott MJ, Aggarwal G, Aitken RJ, et al. Consensus guidelines for perioperative care for Emergency Laparotomy Enhanced Recovery After Surgery (ERAS) Society recommendations part 2—emergency laparotomy: intra and postoperative care. *World J Surgery* 2023;47:1850–80. https://doi.org/10.1007/s00268-023-07020-6

Case 27

Evelyn

Evelyn is an 89-year-old former business woman who now lives in a nursing home. She was sent into the emergency department by ambulance because she was not responding to the nurses, and they were unable to get her to drink anything. She had been coughing and off her food for a day or two and had been seen by the GP who had prescribed some oral antibiotics for a chest infection. She had had many falls over the last year where she had been to the emergency department for head scans and one where she had suffered a femoral neck fracture, leaving her with significant functional impairment. The care home staff thought that Evelyn had lost some weight over the last few months.

Past Medical History

Alzheimer's dementia
Atrial fibrillation
Hip fracture six months ago

Medication

Apixaban 2.5 mg bd	Colecalciferol 800 units od
Donepezil 10 mg od	Furosemide 20 mg od
Loperamide 4 mg od	Sertraline 50 mg od
Simvastatin 40 mg od	

Social History

Evelyn has lived in nursing home for six months following her hip fracture. She transfers with assistance of two and a frame but sometimes gets up unaided and falls. She requires assistance with all activities of daily living and will usually eat when supported by a carer.

Her 'Emergency Health Care Plan' from the care home suggests admission to hospital would be the usual course of action in the event of deterioration that was not responding to community treatment. A 'do not attempt resuscitation' form had been completed.

Her daughter, Sylvia, says that Evelyn has recently been saying to her that she wants to die. This makes Sylvia very upset. Years ago, she had promised her mother that she would never put her in a care home, but the reality was that Evelyn's care needs could not be met in any other way after the hip fracture. She thinks that the care home she chose have provided excellent care for her mother.

Examination

Evelyn was lying curled up on the bed. She looked very thin and had signs of dehydration. Her eyes were closed, and she gave no verbal response but didn't look distressed. Chest clear and no peripheral oedema. Abdomen soft and non-tender. She had a urinary catheter that was inserted in the emergency department for fluid balance monitoring.

Six-Item Screener 0/6

4AT 12/12

BP 112/61 mmHg, pulse 102 bpm, oxygen saturation 92% on air, temperature 36.1°C, weight 43.1 kg, glucose 9.3 mmol/L

Investigations

Biochemistry	Value	Reference range	Haematology	Value	Reference range
Sodium	169	133–146 mmol/L	Haemoglobin	108	115–165 g/L
Potassium	3.9	3.5–5.3 mmol/L	MCV	87	82–100 fL
Urea	27.9	2.5–7.8 mmol/L	White cell count	15.0	4–11 10⁹/L
Creatinine	156	49–90 umol/L	Platelets	179	140–400 10⁹/L
C-reactive protein	21	< 5 mg/L			

Blood tests 12 weeks ago: sodium 144, urea 7.8, creatinine 49
Viral swab for influenza/COVID negative
Chest X-ray—no focal lung lesion
ECG—widespread ST segment depression, sinus rhythm 109–111 bpm

The admitting team identified no acute reversible illness but recognised that she had stopped eating and drinking despite the efforts of the care home staff. She was very severely frail, weak, and dehydrated. Because she had lost weight and generally deteriorated, the medical team thought an underlying cancer was possible. A CT scan of her chest, abdomen, and pelvis was requested. When asked, Sylvia said that she would like 'everything' to be done for her mother.

What is overmedicalisation, and how does it impact frail older people?
Is Evelyn's illness reversible?
When would a palliative approach to her care be best?

How Much Medicine is Too Much?

With increasing capabilities of healthcare systems and increased life expectancy in the developed world over the past century, there has been a significant increase in the expectations placed on healthcare professionals. Returning to being a functioning member of society is commonplace, even after a severe illness. Cure becomes expected. It is not acceptable to society for people to just die. There must be something specific causing death or a failure of treatment before we can accept that this is what is going to happen.

In the political and medical literature, people have recognised this trend of medicalisation of death, and in the early 21st century, there has been a search for an alternative construct. A focus on illness could impair the experience of wellness, and if we ignore what is important to the person seeking help, we may not offer them what they need.

Campaigns such as 'Too Much Medicine' aim to highlight the threats to health and wasted resource from overdiagnosis.[1] This is where increasing rate of diagnosis and medical activity for a particular condition over time does not lead to any recognisable patient benefit. Examples include diagnosing 'conditions' that would never cause symptoms or medicalising ordinary life experiences by changing the diagnostic criteria to include more people in an illness category (even when they might lack symptoms or evidence of benefit from treatment).[2] The overmedicalisation of late life and death can lead to missed opportunities to reduce the burden of futile testing/treating and to focus on what is important to people (often including place of death and time spent with loved ones).

In medicine, it can seem easier to do something because we can. It can be hard to face uncertainty without the reassurance of performing clinical tests or seeking multiple opinions and hard to accept death as part of life. We must also balance against the potential harm of underdiagnosis and undertreatment. In Scotland, the Realistic Medicine programme focusses on delivering person-centred care by undertaking shared decision-making with regards to what tests and treatments to undertake and for what reason.[3] This is not about rationing healthcare to save it for young people, nor is it about adopting a nihilistic approach to caring for old people, but instead, it emphasises prudently utilising medical care as part of attempting to achieve the person's life goals.

Is it 'Reversible'?

Traditionally, people have often been sent to hospital with a 'potentially reversible' illness. It is perceived that an infection can be treatable, a cancer can be curable, and heart failure can be optimised. This is related to the medical model which hospital care was largely designed around. 'The illness is paramount; if we treat the illness, the person will then likely recover'. More than this, it is deeply ingrained through years of medical training that fixing the fixable is always the right thing to do.

Of course, this decontextualised view of the 'crisis' that has led to seeking help omits the vital health trajectory within which the deterioration has occurred. When someone has widespread metastatic cancer and is no longer having any treatments aimed at holding back the progression of their terminal illness, treating an intercurrent infection (the 'reversible pathology') is not going to reverse the situation (N.B. it may well still be the right thing to do). It is less easy to notice this same situation with chronic progressive diseases, and this requires vigilance. Progressive frailty or dementia are common causes of deterioration and death in the UK. With these conditions, recurrent minor illnesses cause a stepwise increase in dependency that should enable us to identify a potentially irreversible situation. Sometimes we can be successful in halting decline, and other times, we cannot.

Palliative and curative approaches are historically quite far apart (one sacrificing the chance of survival for comfort; the other sacrificing comfort for the chance of survival). In geriatrics, there are times for each of these paradigms (although the latter is rarely appropriate for those with very severe frailty), but there is also a wide, and commonly inhabited, middle ground where limited testing, supportive care, and some conservative attempts at treatment co-exist. The twin aims being to focus on comfort and dignity in late life but also giving a chance of recovery—how far to one side or the other is individualised to the person. A combination of the trajectory of decline, degree of frailty, severity of the current illness, and what they think is going to happen can help ascertain where on that spectrum of care you and your patient are most comfortable. If it begins to feel that you might be no longer prolonging life but rather prolonging the dying process, then revisiting the philosophy of treatment is crucial.

What about Evelyn?

Evelyn had been deteriorating towards the end of life for some time. Her progressive cognitive and physical frailty had increased her risk of developing new illnesses and made her less likely to survive them. The six months prior to admission had been difficult for her with inexorable decline in strength and cognition and repeated hospital visits. She had developed very severe frailty (CFS 8). While she had had multiple treatments with curative intent over this time, it became increasingly clear that the situation was irreversible and that a more palliative approach should be considered. Seeking additional causes for her deterioration with imaging studies would not have provided any benefit for Evelyn but merely added to her distress. There may have been an opportunity to approach the final months of her life less medically, reducing medicines and using more careful and detailed advance care planning.

Because of hypoactive delirium superimposed on her dementia, Evelyn couldn't participate in conversations about her care, but Sylvia was involved. Sylvia had felt an enormous amount of guilt when the decision was made to place Evelyn in a care home. This went against a conversation they had had some years before. In her mind, she didn't want to let her mother down again. It was very important that Sylvia received the reassurance that she made good choices for Evelyn and that through her effort and support, her love for her mother had shone through.

When making decisions in Evelyn's best interests alongside Sylvia, the key consideration was 'What would Evelyn have wanted to be done for her if she could see herself now?' Although hard for Sylvia to hear, Evelyn's prior expressed wish to die suggested that she would probably choose a palliative approach to her care. Because Evelyn's recent deterioration was on the background of progressive decline, fixing 'the reversible pathology' was unlikely to have significant impact on her survival; there was no realistic path to 'recovery' for her. It was agreed to make Evelyn's comfort the sole focus of care. It was felt that going back to her care home at that time would be distressing. She died in hospital within the next 24 hours.

Key Points

- 'Reversible pathology' is not a very helpful concept in isolation when treating people with multiple long-term conditions and severe frailty. It is better to consider the wider context of whether this is a 'reversible situation'.
- Understanding the health trajectory of your patient can help to recognise how likely a successful, curative approach to intercurrent illness is and how burdensome the treatments might be to them.
- Avoiding overmedicalisation of late life without adopting a nihilistic approach is a delicate and subtle practice.

Further Reading

1. www.bmj.com/too-much-medicine

2. Aronson JK. When I use a word. . . . Too much healthcare—overdiagnosis. *BMJ* 2022;378:o2062. https://doi.org/10.1136/bmj.o2062

3. *Realistic Medicine—Taking Care: Chief Medical Officer for Scotland Annual Report 2023 to 2024.* https://realisticmedicine.scot/

Zola

Zola is a 90-year-old retired musician who now lives in a care home. Three days ago, she had an unwitnessed fall out of bed. That same day, her carers saw a small amount of red blood in her bowel motions. Today, a large volume of blood was seen in her stool. Bloods tests were sent by the district nurse team. She has an emergency healthcare plan that aims to avoid hospital admission in most situations, unless a reversible cause was suspected. When her blood test results were seen, the out-of-hours GP thought she should be assessed at the hospital. She appeared to be dehydrated, and this sounded reversible. Zola's son and daughter came to hospital with her. They think that she has been drowsier and sleeping more recently. She has fallen twice at the care home in the last month. Fortunately, she did not sustain any injuries, and no further action was required.

Past Medical History

Alzheimer's dementia diagnosed six years ago
Type 2 diabetes
Cardiac pacemaker
Transcatheter aortic valve implantation (TAVI) five years ago
She has a 'do not attempt resuscitation' form and an advance care plan

Medication

Atorvastatin 10 mg od	Clopidogrel 75 mg od
Metformin 500 mg od	Paracetamol 500 mg as required

Social History

Zola lives in a care home. She is no longer mobile and is dependent for all personal care. She has limited speech and dual incontinence.

Examination

Zola is lying on the bed. She appears distressed and intermittently shouts out words that are hard to understand. When her hand was held, she calmed down and said, 'I love you. Please don't go'.

 DOI: 10.1201/9781003582007-28

She has low muscle mass and dry-looking mucus membranes. Her chest is clear and heart sounds normal. There is no peripheral oedema. Her abdomen is soft and non-tender.

Six-Item Screener 0/6

4AT 12/12

BP 122/59 mmHg, pulse 83 bpm, oxygen saturation 92% on air, temperature 37.1°C, weight 44.2kg, glucose 5.1 mmol/L

Investigations

Biochemistry	Value	Reference range	Haematology	Value	Reference range
Sodium	178	133–146 mmol/L	Haemoglobin	135	115–165 g/L
Potassium	3.5	3.5–5.3 mmol/L	MCV˙	83	82–100 fL
Urea	27.9	2.5–7.8 mmol/L	White cell count	13.5	4–11 10⁹/L
Creatinine	168	49–90 umol/L	Neutrophils	11.9	2–7.5 10⁹/L
C-reactive protein	108	< 5 mg/L	Platelets	233	140–400 10⁹/L

Hb_{A1C} 42 mmol/mol two months ago

What is the cause of Zola's rectal bleeding?
What is transcatheter aortic valve implantation?

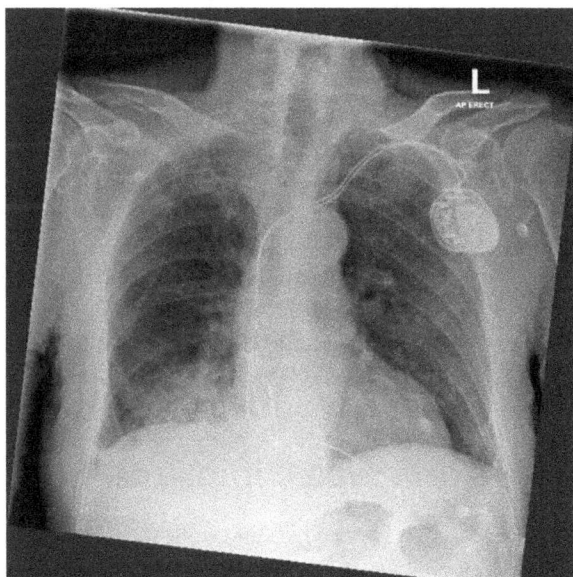

Figure 28.1 Chest X-ray showing cardiac pacemaker, TAVI, and right basal consolidation.

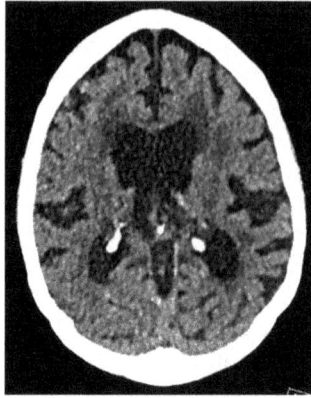

Figure 28.2 Brain CT scan showing atrophy and small vessel ischaemic changes.

Rectal Bleeding

Seeing red blood passed rectally (haematochezia) suggests a source in the large bowel, whereas passing altered blood (i.e. melaena—black and tarry) suggests a source higher up the gastrointestinal (GI) tract. There are several causes of haematochezia that are likely to present in older people with frailty. Diverticular disease is the commonest in developed countries, where more than 60% of people aged over 80 have colonic diverticula.[1] Some people will have episodes of diverticulitis that usually present with left lower quadrant pain and fever. Possible complications of diverticulitis include abscess formation and bowel perforation. Constipation might increase the risk of bleeding. Bleeding episodes are likely to resolve spontaneously. Typical initial management includes treating any associated constipation and withholding blood-thinning mediations.

Angiodysplasia (or vascular ectasia) is caused by degeneration of previously normal blood vessels, which becomes more common in older age. It is also associated with aortic stenosis. Angiodysplasia often causes occult bleeding presenting as iron-deficiency anaemia but can cause haematochezia. Ischaemic colitis is likely to present with abdominal pain and bloody diarrhoea due to impaired blood supply to the large bowel. Bowel cancer more commonly causes occult bleeding than haematochezia. Haemorrhoids can result in low-volume blood loss seen on toilet paper or coating stools. Severe constipation can result in a stercoral ulcer, which is a colonic ulcer caused by hardened, impacted stool leading to ischaemia and necrosis of the bowel wall [see Case 26]. Nicorandil can cause gastrointestinal ulceration, and rarely, rectal ulceration can present as lower GI bleeding. Lower GI endoscopy (i.e. sigmoidoscopy or colonoscopy) can be performed to establish the underlying cause of haematochezia.

Transcatheter Aortic Valve Implantation (TAVI)

Surgical interventions are sometimes appropriate for people with severe aortic stenosis. Typically, this is detected by a combination of symptoms and echocardiography findings.[2] Possible symptoms include shortness of breath, reduced exercise tolerance, angina, syncope, or presyncope. Transthoracic echocardiography criteria define severe aortic stenosis as having at least one of aortic valve area < 1.0 cm^2, peak aortic jet velocity > 4.0 m/s, or mean transthoracic pressure gradient > 40 mmHg.

A TAVI procedure avoids the need for open-heart surgery. A catheter is passed via a femoral artery, and a replacement bioprosthetic valve is inserted, which doesn't require long-term anticoagulation use. TAVI is recommended over surgical aortic valve replacement for people aged over 80 years or with a life expectancy of less than ten years, provided post-TAVI survival is predicted to exceed one year and with a reasonable quality of life.[2] TAVI are easier to implant than surgical valve replacements, but their durability beyond five years is less certain, which is less important for people closer to their end of life. TAVI are associated with lower operative mortality, fewer post-operative complications, and shorter length of stay in hospital compared to surgical procedures. TAVI, compared to no procedure, is associated with lower all-cause mortality and risk of symptomatic heart failure but higher chance of stroke and procedural complications. Very old age, frailty, and multi-morbidity may attenuate any benefit. These factors must be considered on an individual basis using shared decision-making.

What about Zola?

Zola has very severe frailty (CFS 8). In this context, she has developed multiple serious acute health problems. Regardless of any treatments we might offer, she is almost certainly in the last months of life. Recurrent attempts to rescue her in health crisis have been distressing, and her decline has continued. Recognising when it might be the time to prioritise comfort over curative intent and discussing this honestly with loved ones is a key clinical skill in geriatric medicine.

A conversation was had with Zola's son. He was initially confused when it was suggested to him that his mother be admitted to hospital because he thought the advance care plan would keep her out of hospital. The community team had persuaded him that it was necessary after her blood tests results had come back. He thought that his mother had deteriorated a lot in the last month and that the end was approaching. He reflected on his mother's life and the type of person she is. Zola met his father while she was teaching in Sri Lanka, and he was in the army. They had been married for over 60 years and travelled the world together. Before the progression of her dementia, she loved live music and the theatre, did a lot of community work, and was a great socialiser. He felt that Zola would hate to see herself like this. Taking this into account, it was agreed to stop all her regular medications and prescribe 'as required' medicines for symptom control only. Antibiotics and intravenous fluids were not prescribed. The plan was to stop doing blood tests and measuring things like her blood pressure. She was transferred back to the care home, where the staff had always been very kind to her, for end-of-life care.

Key Points

- Diverticular disease is the commonest source of rectal bleeding in older people in developed countries.

- TAVI can improve outcomes of severe aortic stenosis for people who would be unable to have a surgical heart valve replacement.
- Recognising the time to prioritise comfort over curative intent is a key clinical skill in geriatric medicine.

Further Reading

1. Hawkins AT, Wise PE, Chan T, et al. Diverticulitis—an update from the age old paradigm. *Curr Probl Surg* 2020;57:100862. https://doi.org/10.1016/j.cpsurg.2020.100862

2. Otto CM, Nishimura RA, Bonow RO, et al. 2020 ACC/AHA guideline for the management of patients with valvular heart disease. *Circulation* 2021;143:e72–e227. https://doi.org/10.1161/CIR.0000000000000923

Philip

Philip is a 76-year-old man who has been brought into hospital due to being less responsive today. His carers described him as having a grey appearance. Philip is only intermittently answering 'yes' or 'no' to questions. When asked if he was in pain, he nodded and pointed at his catheter. His brother, with whom he lives, has not noticed any cough or shortness of breath. Philip had not had any nausea or vomiting. His oral intake has reduced a little recently. It is unclear when he last opened bowels. He tends to get constipated, and his bowel motions are black in colour. He has had difficulty with painful spasms in his lower abdomen in the past.

Past Medical History

Type 2 diabetes
Ischaemic heart disease
Benign prostatic hyperplasia—long-term urinary catheter for retention of urine
Depression
Sacral pressure damage—under care of the district nursing team

Medication

Amitriptyline 10 mg n	Aspirin 75 mg od
Bisoprolol 10 mg od	Docusate 200 mg bd
Ferrous sulfate 200 mg bd	Gliclazide 80 mg bd
Hyoscine butylbromide 10 mg bd	Oxycodone 5 mg as required
Oxycodone MR 10 mg bd	Paracetamol 1 g qds
Senna 15 mg bd	Sertraline 200 mg od
Tolterodine 2 mg bd	

Intolerance of statins

Social History

Philip has been immobile over the past year. Around the onset, he had a sequence of bad things happen in quick succession. His partner died, he was admitted to hospital with severe cholecystitis, and he had a fall resulting in a knee injury. He now lives with his brother and has carers attending four times a day to assist with all his personal care. He usually sleeps for a lot of the day.

DOI: 10.1201/9781003582007-29

Examination

Philip opens his eyes to speech but has minimal verbal communication. Chest clear, no oedema, abdomen soft and non-tender. Urinary catheter present and draining brown-looking urine. Not able to comply with a detailed neurological examination but is able to move all four limbs against gravity. Grade 3 pressure damage to sacrum.

Six-Item Screener 0/6

4AT 12/12

BP 110/57 mmHg, pulse 89 bpm, oxygen saturation 96% on air, temperature 38.4°C, glucose 7.4 mmol/L, weight 86.3kg

Investigations

Biochemistry	Value	Reference range	Haematology	Value	Reference range
Sodium	138	133–146 mmol/L	Haemoglobin	77	130–180 g/L
Potassium	4.5	3.5–5.3 mmol/L	MCV	84	82–100 fL
Urea	34.0	2.5–7.8 mmol/L	White cell count	22.2	4–11 10^9/L
Creatinine	214	64–104 umol/L	Neutrophils	20.7	2–7.5 10^9/L
C-reactive protein	395	< 5 mg/L	Platelets	381	140–400 10^9/L
Albumin	30	35–50 g/L			

Six months ago: urea 22.1, creatinine 231, haemoglobin 94, Hb_{A1C} 39 mmol/mol (reference range 20–41), ferritin 57.6 ug/L (12–250), vitamin B_{12} 260 ng/L (150–1000), folate 9.1 ug/L (2–18.8)

ECG—left bundle branch block (unchanged from previous ECG), sinus rhythm 93 bpm

Chest X-ray—no abnormality detected

Urine culture grew *Pseudomonas aeruginosa*, which was sensitive to piperacillin-tazobactam.

Progress

Philip was given intravenous fluids and piperacillin-tazobactam for dehydration and a suspected catheter-associated UTI. His oral intake was variable. Over the next few days, he had several episodes of low glucose (< 3.0 mmol/L), leading to receipt of oral glucose gel. He was also given a one-unit blood transfusion.

What is the cause of Philip's anaemia?
Will the pressure ulcer affect his care?
How could his medication be optimised?

Anaemia

Philip has a normocytic anaemia that has been present for more than six months. During this time, his ferritin, vitamin B_{12}, and folate have been in the normal range. His WCC is appropriately raised in response to an infection, and his platelet count is in the normal range, which is against a bone marrow problem, such as myelodysplasia. The anaemia is most likely due to renal impairment, i.e. reduced renal erythropoietin production.

Pressure Ulceration

Pressure ulcers are areas of skin and/or underlying tissue damage usually located beneath bony prominences, such as the sacrum or heels. They are caused by the effects of body weight pressure restricting capillary blood flow that leads to tissue hypoxia and necrosis. Additional factors can include tissue moisture (e.g. incontinence), loss of subcutaneous tissue padding (e.g. frailty and sarcopenia), shear forces created when transferring, and sometimes superimposed infection. The main risk factor is reduced mobility, particularly people who are unable to reposition themselves. This can be longstanding or just occurring around the time of an acute illness, such as a hip fracture. Other important risk factors include cognitive impairment, nutritional deficiency, and loss of sensation. Pressure ulcers are common in hospital and care home settings.

It is important to recognise people at increased risk. Documentation of skin integrity should occur at the time of hospital admission or transfer to a care home. A standard rating scale for pressure ulcers is shown in Figure 29.1. Pressure damage can develop after just a few hours. Repositioning is recommended at least every six hours for people at risk and every four hours for people at high risk.[1] Specialised mattresses should be used that are more able to redistribute pressure. Nutrition should be optimised, and improving mobility is an important goal. Appropriate dressings aim to keep the wound clean and moist. Antibiotics are sometimes required to treat an underlying infection (e.g. osteomyelitis that can be diagnosed by MRI scanning or bone biopsy). Wound swabs are likely to show a mixed growth of surface contaminants and are usually unhelpful. Because of underlying risk factors, pressure ulcers are associated with high mortality, especially when occurring in older people who reside in care homes or when associated with a deep underlying infection.[2]

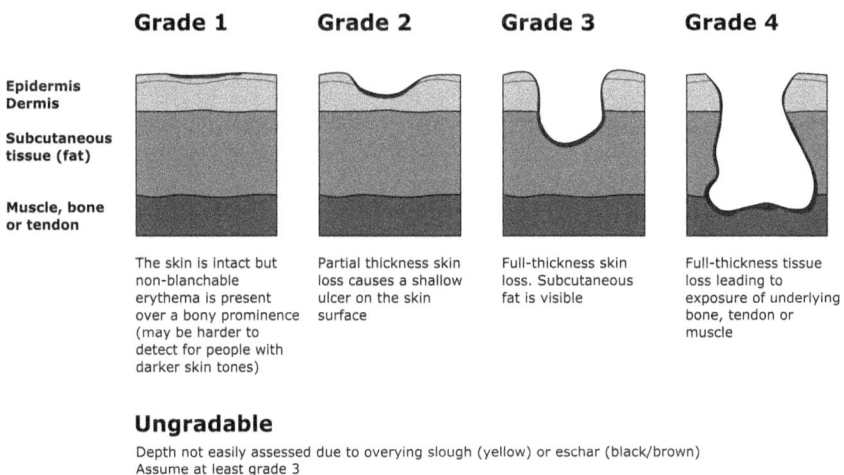

	Grade 1	Grade 2	Grade 3	Grade 4
Epidermis Dermis				
Subcutaneous tissue (fat)				
Muscle, bone or tendon				
	The skin is intact but non-blanchable erythema is present over a bony prominence (may be harder to detect for people with darker skin tones)	Partial thickness skin loss causes a shallow ulcer on the skin surface	Full-thickness skin loss. Subcutaneous fat is visible	Full-thickness tissue loss leading to exposure of underlying bone, tendon or muscle

Ungradable
Depth not easily assessed due to overying slough (yellow) or eschar (black/brown)
Assume at least grade 3

Figure 29.1 Grading of pressure ulcers.

Medication optimisation

Philip currently has delirium due to a catheter-associated UTI. His frailty, multi-morbidity, and polypharmacy all increase his susceptibility to delirium. He is prescribed multiple medications that could be contributing. His anticholinergic burden is very high due to the combination of medications with additive anticholinergic properties (e.g. 'ACB calculator' gives a total score of 11).[3] Reducing this burden is a key component of addressing his delirium.

Philip has complained of crampy lower abdominal pain over the last few months. In case the cause was bladder spasms, he was prescribed tolterodine. When the symptom persisted, he was prescribed hyoscine in case it was due to bowel spasms. He may be constipated, which could also cause crampy abdominal pain. Many of his medications could be constipating, i.e. amitriptyline and tolterodine (anticholinergic), hyoscine (anticholinergic and a specific bowel antispasmodic), ferrous sulfate, and oxycodone. Immobility and his current dehydration also increase the risk of constipation. Docusate is not an effective laxative and should be discontinued. There is no logic in co-prescribing senna to increase bowel contractions and hyoscine to reduce bowel contractions.

Blood tests do not suggest that he is deficient in iron, so ferrous sulfate can be discontinued. It is making his stools black and contributing to constipation. Hyoscine is sometimes prescribed for bowel spasms but is probably no more effective than paracetamol.[4] It has anticholinergic effects but is poorly absorbed from the GI tract, so it may not be an important contributor to his delirium. It should be stopped, at least until his bowels are working. Tolterodine should also be stopped, at least initially. Once his delirium has improved, Philip can be involved in discussions about his future symptom control and the risks/benefits of the available options.

For the last year, Philip has been prescribed amitriptyline and oxycodone for chronic pain since his knee injury. While pain could be a precipitant of delirium, both these medications could adversely affect his cognition. His presentation suggests he has pain related to his catheter, which may improve with antibiotic treatment for the UTI and a change of catheter. There is no clear correct answer. It would be worth considering stopping amitriptyline, at least during his acute illness, and possibly reducing the dose of oxycodone.

Philip's blood glucose has been low during his admission. This may be because he is unwell and has reduced his oral intake during the illness. On the other hand, his Hb_{A1C} was just 39 six months ago, suggesting that he may no longer need medication to control diabetes. Medication requirements can change over time, especially if his diet has changed or he has lost weight. Right now, he is at risk of harm from hypoglycaemia. His gliclazide was withheld, and his blood glucose was monitored.

What about Philip?

Philip has severe frailty (CFS 7). His loss of mobility after the sequence of traumatic events raises the possibility that low mood played a role. After a year of immobility, he will have lost a large amount of muscle strength, and this may be irreversible. He has also developed a pressure ulcer that complicates his recovery and suggests a worse prognosis. Following his acute illness, there is an opportunity to discuss his future goals and consider if any intervention would be useful. Assessment of his mood may also play a role. He is currently prescribed a very high dose of sertraline. Data from clinical studies suggest that an optimal balance between antidepressant efficacy and risk of adverse effects often occurs towards the lower end of the dose range.[5] It may be possible to improve his symptom control through both pharmacological and non-pharmacological changes. Input from the psychiatry team who know him best could help to guide decisions. Once he has recovered from delirium, we can focus on the key question: What does Philip want?

Key Points

- Taking multiple medications with anticholinergic properties can have a cumulative effect.
- Older people with reduced mobility are at a high risk of pressure ulcers. Recognising individual risk, documenting skin damage, and taking preventative measures are important.
- Regular medication review should aim to establish if there is an ongoing benefit, symptomatic or prognostic of each drug.
- Ask your patients, 'What matters to you?'

Further Reading

1. National Institute for Health and Care Excellence. *Pressure Ulcers: Prevention and Management*. 2014. www.nice.org.uk/guidance/cg179

2. Khor HM, Tan J, Saedon NI, et al. Determinants of mortality among older adults with pressure ulcers. *Arch Gerontol Geriatr* 2014;59:536–41. https://doi.org/10.1016/j.archger.2014.07.011

3. www.acbcalc.com

4. Mueller-Lissner S, Tytgat GN, Paulo LG, et al. Placebo- and paracetamol-controlled study on the efficacy and tolerability of hyoscine butylbromide in the treatment of patients with recurrent crampy abdominal pain. *Aliment Pharmacol Ther* 2006;23:1741–8. https://doi.org/10.1111/j.1365–2036.2006.02818.x

5. Furukawa TA, Cipriani A, Cowen PJ, et al. Optimal dose of selective serotonin reuptake inhibitors, venlafaxine, and mirtazapine in major depression: a systematic review and dose-response meta-analysis. *Lancet Psychiatry* 2019;6:601–9. https://doi.org/10.1016/S2215–0366(19)30217–2

Ernie

Ernie is a 90-year-old retired electrician. He came to hospital after a fall at home. He describes catching his foot in the carpet and then falling onto a door frame before landing on the floor on his left side. Since then, he has had pain in his left shoulder, hip, and groin. He didn't have any warning symptoms before falling and doesn't think he lost consciousness. He doesn't think he hit his head and has no back or neck pain. He was feeling well prior to falling.

Past Medical History

Ischaemic heart disease—NSTEMI with percutaneous coronary intervention eight years ago

Implanted cardiac defibrillator (ICD)—deactivated two years ago but pacemaker component still active

Heart failure with reduced ejection fraction (HFrEF; EF 35% eight years ago)

Orthostatic hypotension (OH)—sacubitril/valsartan and spironolactone discontinued six months ago

Alzheimer's dementia diagnosed two years ago

Inguinal hernia repair

'Do not attempt resuscitation' decision

Medication

Allopurinol 100 mg od	Aspirin 75 mg od
Atorvastatin 40 mg od	Bisoprolol 2.5 mg od
Dapagliflozin 10 mg od	Donepezil 10 mg od

Social history

Ernie lives with his wife in a ground floor sheltered accommodation flat. His wife assists him with getting washed and dressed. They do not have any formal care package. He is mobile with a two-wheeled walking frame around their property but doesn't go out without assistance.

 DOI: 10.1201/9781003582007-30

Examination

There were no signs of a head injury and no spinal tenderness. Chest—mild crackles at both bases. Heart sounds reveal a soft systolic murmur. Abdomen soft and non-tender. Left shoulder has no obvious injury and moves okay. Pain on any attempt to move left leg. Good peripheral pulses in both legs.

Six-Item Screener 3/6

4AT 3/12

BP 97/62 mmHg, pulse 71 bpm, oxygen saturation 94% on air, temperature 36.2°C, glucose 4.2 mmol/L, weight 55.1 kg

Investigations

Biochemistry	Value	Reference range	Haematology	Value	Reference range
Sodium	140	133–146 mmol/L	Haemoglobin	145	130–180 g/L
Potassium	4.1	3.5–5.3 mmol/L	MCV	95	82–100 fL
Urea	6.9	2.5–7.8 mmol/L	White cell count	7.1	4–11 10^9/L
Creatinine	102	64–104 umol/L			
C-reactive protein	1	< 5 mg/L	Platelets	178	140–400 10^9/L

ECG—paced rhythm 70 bpm

Preoperative echocardiogram—dilated left ventricle with severely impaired systolic function (EF < 30%). No significant aortic stenosis.

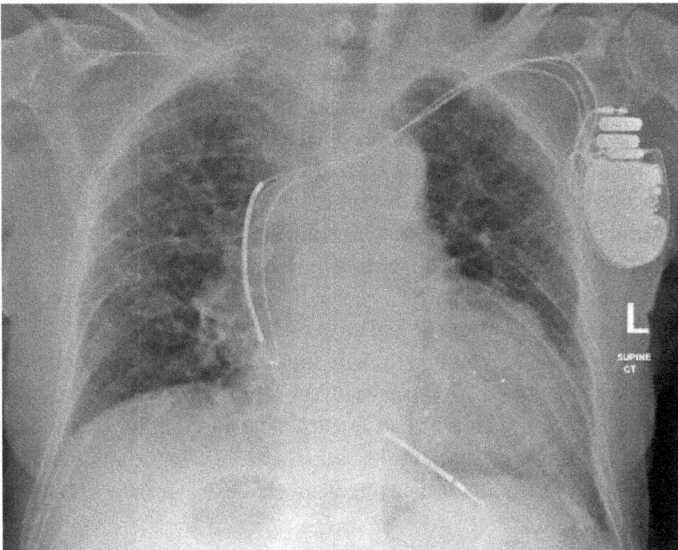

Figure 30.1 Chest X-ray showing an enlarged cardiac silhouette and the ICD.

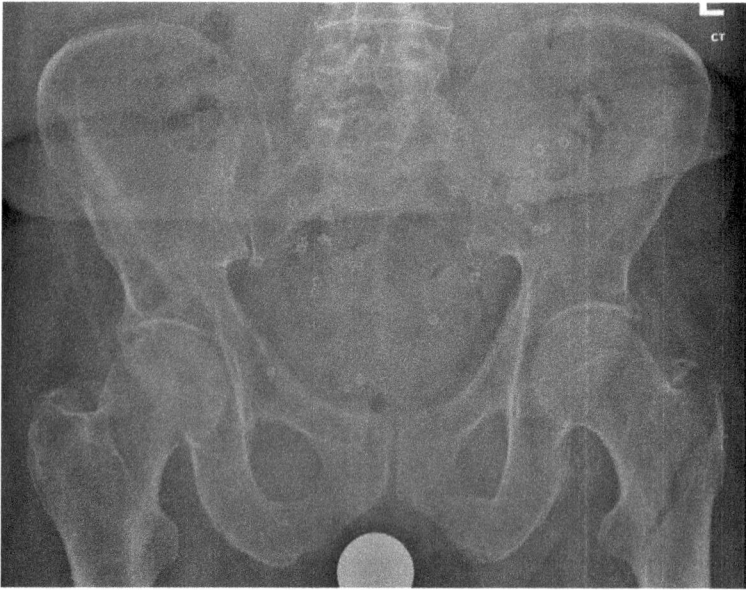

Figure 30.2 Pelvic X-ray showing a left intertrochanteric hip fracture. The metallic spirals are from his prior inguinal hernia surgery.

Progress

Ernie was admitted under the orthopaedic team who fixed his broken hip surgically. A few days later, he was transferred to the geriatric medicine ward to have further rehabilitation. Two weeks later, he had not regained his usual mobility and was only able to transfer from bed to chair with close supervision and the use of a two-wheeled walking frame. Any attempts at walking were limited by low blood pressure and feeling light-headed. Consequently, he spent long periods in bed, which limited his progress. He required a lot of encouragement to even sit out of bed in a chair. Around this time, his BP was in the range 83/52 to 101/52 mmHg. A postural BP measurement found his lying BP to be 94/61, and on standing, this fell to 86/51 mmHg and was associated with feeling light-headed. Compression stockings and an abdominal binder were tried, but neither helped his symptoms nor improved his BP. On examination, his chest was clear, and he had no peripheral oedema.

A discussion was had with Ernie and his wife about discontinuing dapagliflozin due to his symptomatic low blood pressure. His wife is very concerned by this suggestion. When he had been to the cardiology clinic, he had already had to discontinue several tablets due to low blood pressure. The heart specialist had said it was very important that he remain on dapagliflozin because this was an excellent medicine that would protect his heart.

Why did Ernie fall over?
How effective, and how safe, is dapagliflozin for Ernie?

Cause of the Fall

There is a temptation to explain Ernie's fall as a 'simple trip'. He said he caught his foot in the carpet. However, people in good health rarely trip in unhazardous conditions. Ernie has underlying problems that have increased his risk of falling. The mechanism is likely to be multi-factorial. Cognitive impairment can lead people to move too quickly or without the appropriate support or equipment for their degree of physical impairment. He also has a history of OH. Even though he didn't report any preceding symptoms of loss of consciousness, transiently reduced cerebral blood flow could have been a factor in his fall. Some people with OH do not experience typical symptoms but are still at an elevated risk of falling.[1] In addition, some people have amnesia for being unconscious following an episode of syncope.[2] Uncontrolled heart failure could increase the risk of falling, for example, via hypoxia, but Ernie's heart failure seems to be reasonably controlled currently.

Dapagliflozin

Dapagliflozin is a sodium-glucose co-transporter-2 inhibitor (SGLT2i). SGLT2 is a protein found in the proximal tubules of the kidney that reabsorbs glucose and sodium that has been filtered into the urine. SGLT2i block this action, causing the loss of glucose and sodium in the urine, which has a diuretic effect.

Dapagliflozin has been shown to be effective for people with HFrEF. The key clinical trial had a primary outcome measure of a composite of worsening heart failure (defined as a hospitalisation or receiving intravenous therapy for heart failure) or death from a cardiovascular cause.[3] Over an average of 18 months, this primary outcome occurred in 16.3% of people receiving dapagliflozin and 21.2% of people receiving a placebo, giving an absolute risk reduction of 4.9%. So if 20 people with HFrEF receive dapagliflozin for 18 months, one person will avoid either a hospital admission or cardiovascular death, and it will not affect these outcomes for the other 19 people. While this is a statistically significant benefit and at least as effective as many other commonly prescribed medications, these data will not convince everyone that they should take an extra tablet.

In the trial, dapagliflozin was associated with a small reduction in weight (0.7 kg) and systolic BP (1.5 mmHg). Weight loss and BP control may be an additional benefit of dapagliflozin for some people, but Ernie already has a low body mass and BP. Due to the diuretic effect and glycosuria, recognised potential adverse effects of SGLT2i include volume depletion and urinary tract infection (UTI). In the trial, volume depletion was marginally more common with dapagliflozin (7.5% v 6.8%) but UTI was not (0.5% v 0.7%).

But how closely do the trial participants resemble Ernie? The mean age of the people recruited was 66 years. Various trial exclusion criteria would have led to Ernie being judged ineligible to take part. These include having symptomatic hypotension or systolic BP < 95 mmHg, having any non-cardiovascular or renal disease that limits life expectancy to less than two years, and an inability to understand and/or comply with study medication and procedures. Nobody like Ernie was recruited to the trial. Frailty is a state of vulnerability caused by biological ageing and is associated with an increased risk of harm from stressors, including medication-related harm.[4] The result is that we neither know the chance that

Ernie will benefit from dapagliflozin or the risk of harm to him. This hampers our ability to effectively practice shared decision-making. It is important that we acknowledge this uncertainty in our discussions. Extrapolating the results achieved in different groups of people is not the same as practicing evidence-based medicine.

What about Ernie?

Ernie has a complex mix of physical and cognitive co-morbidities and had moderate frailty prior to admission (CFS 6). The extent of his recovery from the hip fracture is uncertain currently. It is likely that he is in the last year of his life. With his input, a prior decision was made to deactivate his ICD. This placed the emphasis on symptom control rather than therapies that could prolong his life.

Healthcare professionals can find it challenging to discuss the risks and benefits of medications with patients. In part, this is due to uncertain knowledge. Clinical trials, often sponsored by pharmaceutical companies, recruit highly selected groups of patients. It can be hard to know if the trial findings are likely to be replicated for the person you are treating. Outcome data can be presented in less comprehensible ways, such as relative risk reduction. We tend to overestimate benefits.[5] In addition, making informed decisions requires weighing up a large amount of information. This necessitates a degree of health literacy that not every patient has.

Dapagliflozin has a diuretic effect, and this could help with symptoms of heart failure, but it is also likely to contribute to low BP and his risk of falling. Ernie is also prescribed bisoprolol, which tends to only have a small effect on supine BP. He has a pacemaker that prevents bradycardia, but bisoprolol may impair the normal physiological heart rate increase in response to postural change. Other therapies have failed to resolve this problem, and he is not making progress with rehabilitation. A discussion was had to explore the potential risks and benefit of both dapagliflozin and bisoprolol with Ernie and his wife. It was agreed that the most important goal was to try to get Ernie mobile again so that he could return to living with his wife. It was felt that bisoprolol was less likely to be causing his OH and could be beneficial for his heart failure, so this was continued. Dapagliflozin was deprescribed. Should his OH continue, then the bisoprolol could be revisited. Should he develop symptomatic heart failure, then that may also need further medication adjustments.

Key Points

- OH can contribute to the mechanism of falls even for people who do not report light-headedness or transient loss of consciousness.
- Selection criteria for clinical trials can make it hard to know if the person you are treating will have similar risks and benefits.
- Even for effective therapies, the actual number needed to treat can be high, i.e. most people prescribed the medicine won't benefit from treatment.
- Limited life expectancy and increased vulnerability associated with frailty sometimes make deprescribing an option that better aligns with patient goals.

Further Reading

1. Claffey P, Pérez-Denia L, Lavan A, et al. Asymptomatic orthostatic hypotension and risk of falls in community-dwelling older people. *Age Ageing* 2022;51:1–8. https://doi.org/10.1093/ageing/afac295

2. O'Dwyer C, Bennett K, Langan Y, et al. Amnesia for loss of consciousness is common in vasovagal syncope. *EP Europace* 2011;13:1040–5. https://doi.org/10.1093/europace/eur069

3. McMurray JJV, Solomon SD, Inzucchi SE, et al. Dapagliflozin in patients with heart failure and reduced ejection fraction. *N Engl J Med* 2019;381:1995–2008. https://doi.org/10.1056/NEJMoa1911303

4. Lam JYJ, Barras M, Scott IA, et al. Scoping review of studies evaluating frailty and its association with medication harm. *Drugs Aging* 2022;39:333–53. https://doi.org/10.1007/s40266-022-00940-3

5. Treadwell JS, Wong G, Milburn-Curtis C, et al. GPs' understanding of the benefits and harms of treatments for long-term conditions: an online survey. *BJGP Open* 2020. https://doi.org/10.3399/bjgpopen20X101016

Index

Note: Page numbers in *italics* indicate a figure and page numbers in **bold** indicate a table on the corresponding page.

For Product Safety Concerns and Information please contact our EU
representative GPSR@taylorandfrancis.com
Taylor & Francis Verlag GmbH, Kaufingerstraße 24, 80331 München, Germany